Mometrix
TEST PREPARATION

CHFM®

Exam Secrets Study Guide

Dear Future Exam Success Story

First of all, **THANK YOU** for purchasing Mometrix study materials!

Second, congratulations! You are one of the few determined test-takers who are committed to doing whatever it takes to excel on your exam. **You have come to the right place.** We developed these study materials with one goal in mind: to deliver you the information you need in a format that's concise and easy to use.

In addition to optimizing your guide for the content of the test, we've outlined our recommended steps for breaking down the preparation process into small, attainable goals so you can make sure you stay on track.

We've also analyzed the entire test-taking process, identifying the most common pitfalls and showing how you can overcome them and be ready for any curveball the test throws you.

Standardized testing is one of the biggest obstacles on your road to success, which only increases the importance of doing well in the high-pressure, high-stakes environment of test day. Your results on this test could have a significant impact on your future, and this guide provides the information and practical advice to help you achieve your full potential on test day.

Your success is our success

We would love to hear from you! If you would like to share the story of your exam success or if you have any questions or comments in regard to our products, please contact us at **800-673-8175** or **support@mometrix.com**.

Thanks again for your business and we wish you continued success!

Sincerely,
The Mometrix Test Preparation Team

Need more help? Check out our flashcards at:
http://MometrixFlashcards.com/CHFM

Written and edited by the Mometrix Exam Secrets Test Prep Team
Printed in the United States of America

TABLE OF CONTENTS

Introduction

Thank you for purchasing this resource! You have made the choice to prepare yourself for a test that could have a huge impact on your future, and this guide is designed to help you be fully ready for test day. Obviously, it's important to have a solid understanding of the test material, but you also need to be prepared for the unique environment and stressors of the test, so that you can perform to the best of your abilities.

For this purpose, the first section that appears in this guide is the **Secret Keys**. We've devoted countless hours to meticulously researching what works and what doesn't, and we've boiled down our findings to the five most impactful steps you can take to improve your performance on the test. We start at the beginning with study planning and move through the preparation process, all the way to the testing strategies that will help you get the most out of what you know when you're finally sitting in front of the test.

We recommend that you start preparing for your test as far in advance as possible. However, if you've bought this guide as a last-minute study resource and only have a few days before your test, we recommend that you skip over the first two Secret Keys since they address a long-term study plan.

If you struggle with **test anxiety**, we strongly encourage you to check out our recommendations for how you can overcome it. Test anxiety is a formidable foe, but it can be beaten, and we want to make sure you have the tools you need to defeat it.

Secret Key 1: Plan Big, Study Small

There's a lot riding on your performance. If you want to ace this test, you're going to need to keep your skills sharp and the material fresh in your mind. You need a plan that lets you review everything you need to know while still fitting in your schedule. We'll break this strategy down into three categories.

Information Organization

Start with the information you already have: the official test outline. From this, you can make a complete list of all the concepts you need to cover before the test. Organize these concepts into groups that can be studied together, and create a list of any related vocabulary you need to learn so you can brush up on any difficult terms. You'll want to keep this vocabulary list handy once you actually start studying since you may need to add to it along the way.

Time Management

Once you have your set of study concepts, decide how to spread them out over the time you have left before the test. Break your study plan into small, clear goals so you have a manageable task for each day and know exactly what you're doing. Then just focus on one small step at a time. When you manage your time this way, you don't need to spend hours at a time studying. Studying a small block of content for a short period each day helps you retain information better and avoid stressing over how much you have left to do. You can relax knowing that you have a plan to cover everything in time. In order for this strategy to be effective though, you have to start studying early and stick to your schedule. Avoid the exhaustion and futility that comes from last-minute cramming!

Study Environment

The environment you study in has a big impact on your learning. Studying in a coffee shop, while probably more enjoyable, is not likely to be as fruitful as studying in a quiet room. It's important to keep distractions to a minimum. You're only planning to study for a short block of time, so make the most of it. Don't pause to check your phone or get up to find a snack. It's also important to **avoid multitasking**. Research has consistently shown that multitasking will make your studying dramatically less effective. Your study area should also be comfortable and well-lit so you don't have the distraction of straining your eyes or sitting on an uncomfortable chair.

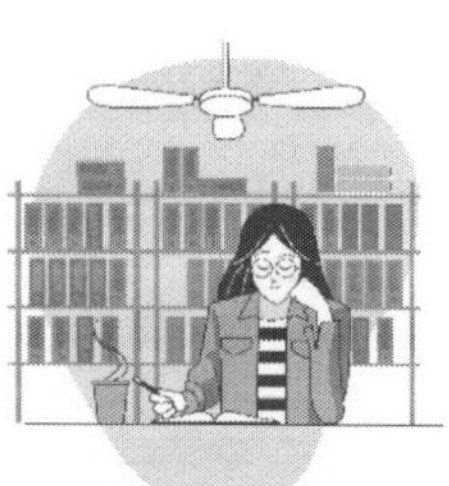

The time of day you study is also important. You want to be rested and alert. Don't wait until just before bedtime. Study when you'll be most likely to comprehend and remember. Even better, if you know what time of day your test will be, set that time aside for study. That way your brain will be used to working on that subject at that specific time and you'll have a better chance of recalling information.

Finally, it can be helpful to team up with others who are studying for the same test. Your actual studying should be done in as isolated an environment as possible, but the work of organizing the information and setting up the study plan can be divided up. In between study sessions, you can discuss with your teammates the concepts that you're all studying and quiz each other on the details. Just be sure that your teammates are as serious about the test as you are. If you find that your study time is being replaced with social time, you might need to find a new team.

Secret Key 2: Make Your Studying Count

You're devoting a lot of time and effort to preparing for this test, so you want to be absolutely certain it will pay off. This means doing more than just reading the content and hoping you can remember it on test day. It's important to make every minute of study count. There are two main areas you can focus on to make your studying count.

Retention

It doesn't matter how much time you study if you can't remember the material. You need to make sure you are retaining the concepts. To check your retention of the information you're learning, try recalling it at later times with minimal prompting. Try carrying around flashcards and glance at one or two from time to time or ask a friend who's also studying for the test to quiz you.

To enhance your retention, look for ways to put the information into practice so that you can apply it rather than simply recalling it. If you're using the information in practical ways, it will be much easier to remember. Similarly, it helps to solidify a concept in your mind if you're not only reading it to yourself but also explaining it to someone else. Ask a friend to let you teach them about a concept you're a little shaky on (or speak aloud to an imaginary audience if necessary). As you try to summarize, define, give examples, and answer your friend's questions, you'll understand the concepts better and they will stay with you longer. Finally, step back for a big picture view and ask yourself how each piece of information fits with the whole subject. When you link the different concepts together and see them working together as a whole, it's easier to remember the individual components.

Finally, practice showing your work on any multi-step problems, even if you're just studying. Writing out each step you take to solve a problem will help solidify the process in your mind, and you'll be more likely to remember it during the test.

Modality

Modality simply refers to the means or method by which you study. Choosing a study modality that fits your own individual learning style is crucial. No two people learn best in exactly the same way, so it's important to know your strengths and use them to your advantage.

For example, if you learn best by visualization, focus on visualizing a concept in your mind and draw an image or a diagram. Try color-coding your notes, illustrating them, or creating symbols that will trigger your mind to recall a learned concept. If you learn best by hearing or discussing information, find a study partner who learns the same way or read aloud to yourself. Think about how to put the information in your own words. Imagine that you are giving a lecture on the topic and record yourself so you can listen to it later.

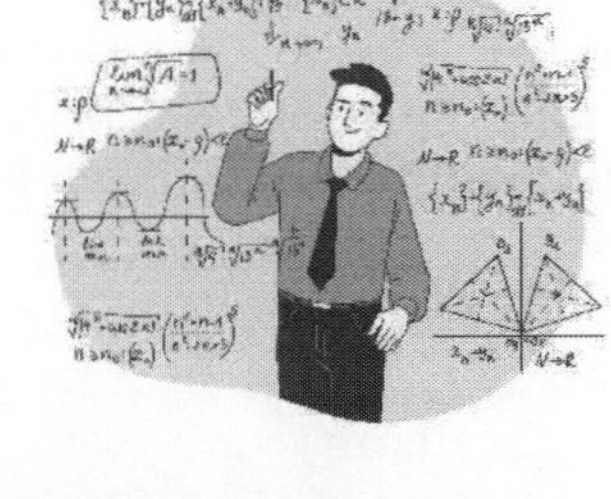

For any learning style, flashcards can be helpful. Organize the information so you can take advantage of spare moments to review. Underline key words or phrases. Use different colors for different categories. Mnemonic devices (such as creating a short list in which every item starts with the same letter) can also help with retention. Find what works best for you and use it to store the information in your mind most effectively and easily.

Secret Key 3: Practice the Right Way

Your success on test day depends not only on how many hours you put into preparing, but also on whether you prepared the right way. It's good to check along the way to see if your studying is paying off. One of the most effective ways to do this is by taking practice tests to evaluate your progress. Practice tests are useful because they show exactly where you need to improve. Every time you take a practice test, pay special attention to these three groups of questions:

- The questions you got wrong
- The questions you had to guess on, even if you guessed right
- The questions you found difficult or slow to work through

This will show you exactly what your weak areas are, and where you need to devote more study time. Ask yourself why each of these questions gave you trouble. Was it because you didn't understand the material? Was it because you didn't remember the vocabulary? Do you need more repetitions on this type of question to build speed and confidence? Dig into those questions and figure out how you can strengthen your weak areas as you go back to review the material.

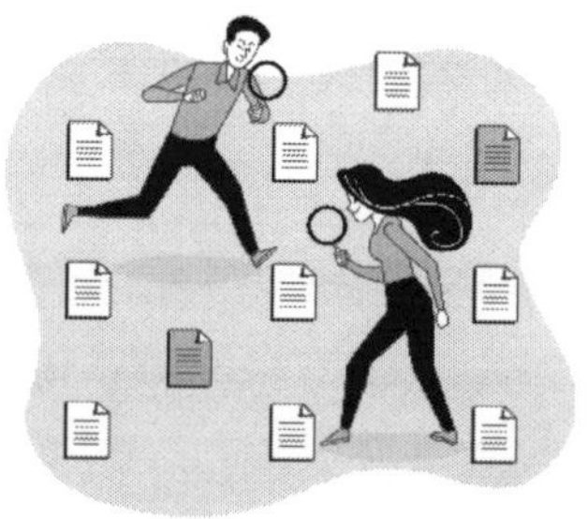

Additionally, many practice tests have a section explaining the answer choices. It can be tempting to read the explanation and think that you now have a good understanding of the concept. However, an explanation likely only covers part of the question's broader context. Even if the explanation makes perfect sense, **go back and investigate** every concept related to the question until you're positive you have a thorough understanding.

As you go along, keep in mind that the practice test is just that: practice. Memorizing these questions and answers will not be very helpful on the actual test because it is unlikely to have any of the same exact questions. If you only know the right answers to the sample questions, you won't be prepared for the real thing. **Study the concepts** until you understand them fully, and then you'll be able to answer any question that shows up on the test.

It's important to wait on the practice tests until you're ready. If you take a test on your first day of study, you may be overwhelmed by the amount of material covered and how much you need to learn. Work up to it gradually.

On test day, you'll need to be prepared for answering questions, managing your time, and using the test-taking strategies you've learned. It's a lot to balance, like a mental marathon that will have a big impact on your future. Like training for a marathon, you'll need to start slowly and work your way up. When test day arrives, you'll be ready.

Start with the strategies you've read in the first two Secret Keys—plan your course and study in the way that works best for you. If you have time, consider using multiple study resources to get different approaches to the same concepts. It can be helpful to see difficult concepts from more than one angle. Then find a good source for practice tests. Many times, the test website will suggest potential study resources or provide sample tests.

Practice Test Strategy

If you're able to find at least three practice tests, we recommend this strategy:

UNTIMED AND OPEN-BOOK PRACTICE

Take the first test with no time constraints and with your notes and study guide handy. Take your time and focus on applying the strategies you've learned.

TIMED AND OPEN-BOOK PRACTICE

Take the second practice test open-book as well, but set a timer and practice pacing yourself to finish in time.

TIMED AND CLOSED-BOOK PRACTICE

Take any other practice tests as if it were test day. Set a timer and put away your study materials. Sit at a table or desk in a quiet room, imagine yourself at the testing center, and answer questions as quickly and accurately as possible.

Keep repeating timed and closed-book tests on a regular basis until you run out of practice tests or it's time for the actual test. Your mind will be ready for the schedule and stress of test day, and you'll be able to focus on recalling the material you've learned.

Secret Key 4: Pace Yourself

Once you're fully prepared for the material on the test, your biggest challenge on test day will be managing your time. Just knowing that the clock is ticking can make you panic even if you have plenty of time left. Work on pacing yourself so you can build confidence against the time constraints of the exam. Pacing is a difficult skill to master, especially in a high-pressure environment, so **practice is vital**.

Set time expectations for your pace based on how much time is available. For example, if a section has 60 questions and the time limit is 30 minutes, you know you have to average 30 seconds or less per question in order to answer them all. Although 30 seconds is the hard limit, set 25 seconds per question as your goal, so you reserve extra time to spend on harder questions. When you budget extra time for the harder questions, you no longer have any reason to stress when those questions take longer to answer.

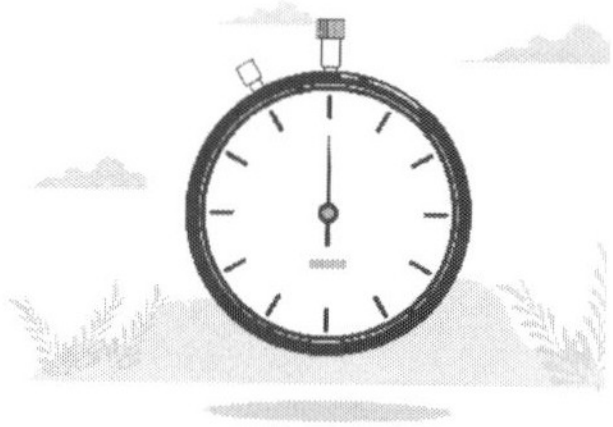

Don't let this time expectation distract you from working through the test at a calm, steady pace, but keep it in mind so you don't spend too much time on any one question. Recognize that taking extra time on one question you don't understand may keep you from answering two that you do understand later in the test. If your time limit for a question is up and you're still not sure of the answer, mark it and move on, and come back to it later if the time and the test format allow. If the testing format doesn't allow you to return to earlier questions, just make an educated guess; then put it out of your mind and move on.

On the easier questions, be careful not to rush. It may seem wise to hurry through them so you have more time for the challenging ones, but it's not worth missing one if you know the concept and just didn't take the time to read the question fully. Work efficiently but make sure you understand the question and have looked at all of the answer choices, since more than one may seem right at first.

Even if you're paying attention to the time, you may find yourself a little behind at some point. You should speed up to get back on track, but do so wisely. Don't panic; just take a few seconds less on each question until you're caught up. Don't guess without thinking, but do look through the answer choices and eliminate any you know are wrong. If you can get down to two choices, it is often worthwhile to guess from those. Once you've chosen an answer, move on and don't dwell on any that you skipped or had to hurry through. If a question was taking too long, chances are it was one of the harder ones, so you weren't as likely to get it right anyway.

On the other hand, if you find yourself getting ahead of schedule, it may be beneficial to slow down a little. The more quickly you work, the more likely you are to make a careless mistake that will affect your score. You've budgeted time for each question, so don't be afraid to spend that time. Practice an efficient but careful pace to get the most out of the time you have.

Secret Key 5: Have a Plan for Guessing

When you're taking the test, you may find yourself stuck on a question. Some of the answer choices seem better than others, but you don't see the one answer choice that is obviously correct. What do you do?

The scenario described above is very common, yet most test takers have not effectively prepared for it. Developing and practicing a plan for guessing may be one of the single most effective uses of your time as you get ready for the exam.

In developing your plan for guessing, there are three questions to address:

- When should you start the guessing process?
- How should you narrow down the choices?
- Which answer should you choose?

When to Start the Guessing Process

Unless your plan for guessing is to select C every time (which, despite its merits, is not what we recommend), you need to leave yourself enough time to apply your answer elimination strategies. Since you have a limited amount of time for each question, that means that if you're going to give yourself the best shot at guessing correctly, you have to decide quickly whether or not you will guess.

Of course, the best-case scenario is that you don't have to guess at all, so first, see if you can answer the question based on your knowledge of the subject and basic reasoning skills. Focus on the key words in the question and try to jog your memory of related topics. Give yourself a chance to bring the knowledge to mind, but once you realize that you don't have (or you can't access) the knowledge you need to answer the question, it's time to start the guessing process.

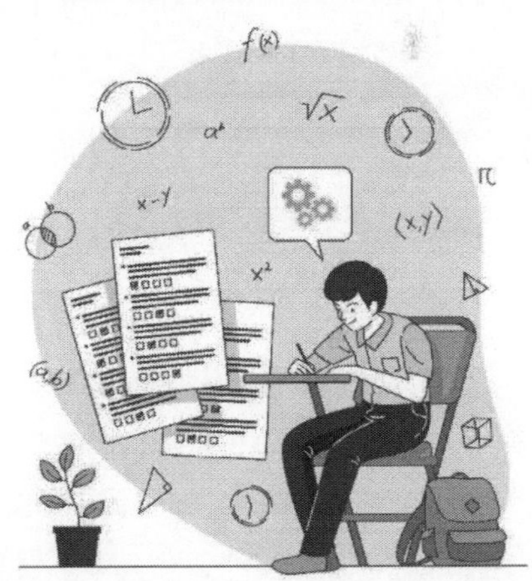

It's almost always better to start the guessing process too early than too late. It only takes a few seconds to remember something and answer the question from knowledge. Carefully eliminating wrong answer choices takes longer. Plus, going through the process of eliminating answer choices can actually help jog your memory.

Summary: Start the guessing process as soon as you decide that you can't answer the question based on your knowledge.

How to Narrow Down the Choices

The next chapter in this book (**Test-Taking Strategies**) includes a wide range of strategies for how to approach questions and how to look for answer choices to eliminate. You will definitely want to read those carefully, practice them, and figure out which ones work best for you. Here though, we're going to address a mindset rather than a particular strategy.

Your odds of guessing an answer correctly depend on how many options you are choosing from.

Number of options left	5	4	3	2	1
Odds of guessing correctly	20%	25%	33%	50%	100%

You can see from this chart just how valuable it is to be able to eliminate incorrect answers and make an educated guess, but there are two things that many test takers do that cause them to miss out on the benefits of guessing:

- Accidentally eliminating the correct answer
- Selecting an answer based on an impression

We'll look at the first one here, and the second one in the next section.

To avoid accidentally eliminating the correct answer, we recommend a thought exercise called **the $5 challenge**. In this challenge, you only eliminate an answer choice from contention if you are willing to bet $5 on it being wrong. Why $5? Five dollars is a small but not insignificant amount of money. It's an amount you could afford to lose but wouldn't want to throw away. And while losing $5 once might not hurt too much, doing it twenty times will set you back $100. In the same way, each small decision you make—eliminating a choice here, guessing on a question there—won't by itself impact your score very much, but when you put them all together, they can make a big difference. By holding each answer choice elimination decision to a higher standard, you can reduce the risk of accidentally eliminating the correct answer.

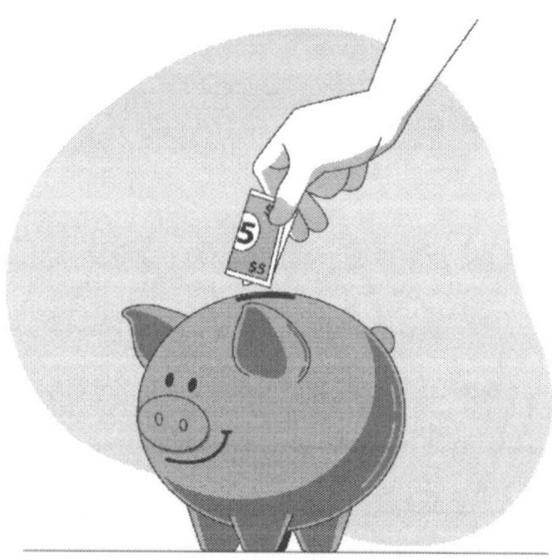

The $5 challenge can also be applied in a positive sense: If you are willing to bet $5 that an answer choice *is* correct, go ahead and mark it as correct.

Summary: Only eliminate an answer choice if you are willing to bet $5 that it is wrong.

Which Answer to Choose

You're taking the test. You've run into a hard question and decided you'll have to guess. You've eliminated all the answer choices you're willing to bet $5 on. Now you have to pick an answer. Why do we even need to talk about this? Why can't you just pick whichever one you feel like when the time comes?

The answer to these questions is that if you don't come into the test with a plan, you'll rely on your impression to select an answer choice, and if you do that, you risk falling into a trap. The test writers know that everyone who takes their test will be guessing on some of the questions, so they intentionally write wrong answer choices to seem plausible. You still have to pick an answer though, and if the wrong answer choices are designed to look right, how can you ever be sure that you're not falling for their trap? The best solution we've found to this dilemma is to take the decision out of your hands entirely. Here is the process we recommend:

Once you've eliminated any choices that you are confident (willing to bet $5) are wrong, select the first remaining choice as your answer.

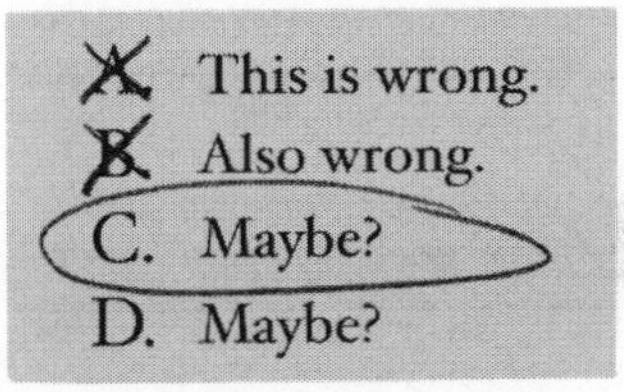

Whether you choose to select the first remaining choice, the second, or the last, the important thing is that you use some preselected standard. Using this approach guarantees that you will not be enticed into selecting an answer choice that looks right, because you are not basing your decision on how the answer choices look.

This is not meant to make you question your knowledge. Instead, it is to help you recognize the difference between your knowledge and your impressions. There's a huge difference between thinking an answer is right because of what you know, and thinking an answer is right because it looks or sounds like it should be right.

Summary: To ensure that your selection is appropriately random, make a predetermined selection from among all answer choices you have not eliminated.

Test-Taking Strategies

This section contains a list of test-taking strategies that you may find helpful as you work through the test. By taking what you know and applying logical thought, you can maximize your chances of answering any question correctly!

It is very important to realize that every question is different and every person is different: no single strategy will work on every question, and no single strategy will work for every person. That's why we've included all of them here, so you can try them out and determine which ones work best for different types of questions and which ones work best for you.

Question Strategies

☑ Read Carefully

Read the question and the answer choices carefully. Don't miss the question because you misread the terms. You have plenty of time to read each question thoroughly and make sure you understand what is being asked. Yet a happy medium must be attained, so don't waste too much time. You must read carefully and efficiently.

☑ Contextual Clues

Look for contextual clues. If the question includes a word you are not familiar with, look at the immediate context for some indication of what the word might mean. Contextual clues can often give you all the information you need to decipher the meaning of an unfamiliar word. Even if you can't determine the meaning, you may be able to narrow down the possibilities enough to make a solid guess at the answer to the question.

☑ Prefixes

If you're having trouble with a word in the question or answer choices, try dissecting it. Take advantage of every clue that the word might include. Prefixes can be a huge help. Usually, they allow you to determine a basic meaning. *Pre-* means before, *post-* means after, *pro-* is positive, *de-* is negative. From prefixes, you can get an idea of the general meaning of the word and try to put it into context.

☑ Hedge Words

Watch out for critical hedge words, such as *likely, may, can, often, almost, mostly, usually, generally, rarely,* and *sometimes*. Question writers insert these hedge phrases to cover every possibility. Often an answer choice will be wrong simply because it leaves no room for exception. Be on guard for answer choices that have definitive words such as *exactly* and *always*.

☑ Switchback Words

Stay alert for *switchbacks*. These are the words and phrases frequently used to alert you to shifts in thought. The most common switchback words are *but, although,* and *however*. Others include *nevertheless, on the other hand, even though, while, in spite of, despite,* and *regardless of*. Switchback words are important to catch because they can change the direction of the question or an answer choice.

✅ Face Value

When in doubt, use common sense. Accept the situation in the problem at face value. Don't read too much into it. These problems will not require you to make wild assumptions. If you have to go beyond creativity and warp time or space in order to have an answer choice fit the question, then you should move on and consider the other answer choices. These are normal problems rooted in reality. The applicable relationship or explanation may not be readily apparent, but it is there for you to figure out. Use your common sense to interpret anything that isn't clear.

Answer Choice Strategies

✅ Answer Selection

The most thorough way to pick an answer choice is to identify and eliminate wrong answers until only one is left, then confirm it is the correct answer. Sometimes an answer choice may immediately seem right, but be careful. The test writers will usually put more than one reasonable answer choice on each question, so take a second to read all of them and make sure that the other choices are not equally obvious. As long as you have time left, it is better to read every answer choice than to pick the first one that looks right without checking the others.

✅ Answer Choice Families

An answer choice family consists of two (in rare cases, three) answer choices that are very similar in construction and cannot all be true at the same time. If you see two answer choices that are direct opposites or parallels, one of them is usually the correct answer. For instance, if one answer choice says that quantity x increases and another either says that quantity x decreases (opposite) or says that quantity y increases (parallel), then those answer choices would fall into the same family. An answer choice that doesn't match the construction of the answer choice family is more likely to be incorrect. Most questions will not have answer choice families, but when they do appear, you should be prepared to recognize them.

✅ Eliminate Answers

Eliminate answer choices as soon as you realize they are wrong, but make sure you consider all possibilities. If you are eliminating answer choices and realize that the last one you are left with is also wrong, don't panic. Start over and consider each choice again. There may be something you missed the first time that you will realize on the second pass.

✅ Avoid Fact Traps

Don't be distracted by an answer choice that is factually true but doesn't answer the question. You are looking for the choice that answers the question. Stay focused on what the question is asking for so you don't accidentally pick an answer that is true but incorrect. Always go back to the question and make sure the answer choice you've selected actually answers the question and is not merely a true statement.

✅ Extreme Statements

In general, you should avoid answers that put forth extreme actions as standard practice or proclaim controversial ideas as established fact. An answer choice that states the "process should be used in certain situations, if..." is much more likely to be correct than one that states the "process should be discontinued completely." The first is a calm rational statement and doesn't even make a definitive, uncompromising stance, using a hedge word *if* to provide wiggle room, whereas the second choice is far more extreme.

⊘ BENCHMARK

As you read through the answer choices and you come across one that seems to answer the question well, mentally select that answer choice. This is not your final answer, but it's the one that will help you evaluate the other answer choices. The one that you selected is your benchmark or standard for judging each of the other answer choices. Every other answer choice must be compared to your benchmark. That choice is correct until proven otherwise by another answer choice beating it. If you find a better answer, then that one becomes your new benchmark. Once you've decided that no other choice answers the question as well as your benchmark, you have your final answer.

⊘ PREDICT THE ANSWER

Before you even start looking at the answer choices, it is often best to try to predict the answer. When you come up with the answer on your own, it is easier to avoid distractions and traps because you will know exactly what to look for. The right answer choice is unlikely to be word-for-word what you came up with, but it should be a close match. Even if you are confident that you have the right answer, you should still take the time to read each option before moving on.

General Strategies

⊘ TOUGH QUESTIONS

If you are stumped on a problem or it appears too hard or too difficult, don't waste time. Move on! Remember though, if you can quickly check for obviously incorrect answer choices, your chances of guessing correctly are greatly improved. Before you completely give up, at least try to knock out a couple of possible answers. Eliminate what you can and then guess at the remaining answer choices before moving on.

⊘ CHECK YOUR WORK

Since you will probably not know every term listed and the answer to every question, it is important that you get credit for the ones that you do know. Don't miss any questions through careless mistakes. If at all possible, try to take a second to look back over your answer selection and make sure you've selected the correct answer choice and haven't made a costly careless mistake (such as marking an answer choice that you didn't mean to mark). This quick double check should more than pay for itself in caught mistakes for the time it costs.

⊘ PACE YOURSELF

It's easy to be overwhelmed when you're looking at a page full of questions; your mind is confused and full of random thoughts, and the clock is ticking down faster than you would like. Calm down and maintain the pace that you have set for yourself. Especially as you get down to the last few minutes of the test, don't let the small numbers on the clock make you panic. As long as you are on track by monitoring your pace, you are guaranteed to have time for each question.

⊘ DON'T RUSH

It is very easy to make errors when you are in a hurry. Maintaining a fast pace in answering questions is pointless if it makes you miss questions that you would have gotten right otherwise. Test writers like to include distracting information and wrong answers that seem right. Taking a little extra time to avoid careless mistakes can make all the difference in your test score. Find a pace that allows you to be confident in the answers that you select.

⊘ KEEP MOVING

Panicking will not help you pass the test, so do your best to stay calm and keep moving. Taking deep breaths and going through the answer elimination steps you practiced can help to break through a stress barrier and keep your pace.

Final Notes

The combination of a solid foundation of content knowledge and the confidence that comes from practicing your plan for applying that knowledge is the key to maximizing your performance on test day. As your foundation of content knowledge is built up and strengthened, you'll find that the strategies included in this chapter become more and more effective in helping you quickly sift through the distractions and traps of the test to isolate the correct answer.

Now that you're preparing to move forward into the test content chapters of this book, be sure to keep your goal in mind. As you read, think about how you will be able to apply this information on the test. If you've already seen sample questions for the test and you have an idea of the question format and style, try to come up with questions of your own that you can answer based on what you're reading. This will give you valuable practice applying your knowledge in the same ways you can expect to on test day.

Good luck and good studying!

Why Certify?

CHFM: Certified Healthcare Facility Manager

- Raise the standards in your field and distinguish your experience.
- Use your credentials to further your career.
- Improve your skills and abilities to manage workers

Candidate Handbook

http://www.aha.org/certifcenter/CHFM/index.shtml

Score

Scores are reported in written form only, in person or by US mail. Scores are not reported over the telephone, by electronic mail or by fax.

The score report indicates a "Pass" or "Fail." Raw score on the total examination determines Pass/Fail status. Additional detail is provided in the form of raw scores by major categories of the examination content outline. A raw score is the number of items answered correctly. Even though the examination consists of 110 items, the score is based on 100 items. Ten (10) items are "pretest" items and do not affect the candidate's score.

Compliance

Occupancy Codes

Occupancy codes are standards, rules, and regulations established by state and local government agencies to ensure buildings are safe and properly constructed. Occupancy codes outline acceptable levels of sanitation, health, life safety, and fire preparedness in healthcare facilities. The CHFM must maintain the occupancy codes in each building he/she manages, so the buildings can be legally occupied and used. Details of the codes vary according to government jurisdiction. Government officials may conduct periodic inspections of a building and its specific equipment, or may require the occupants to do so. Electrical switches and fire protection equipment are tested at regular intervals to ensure they are in good working order. If the government finds noncompliance during an inspection, then it issues a warning and may revoke the certificate of occupancy if the situation is not corrected. Structural noncompliance means the building can be condemned and demolished.

Inspection of Fire Protection System

Fire protection equipment is rarely used, so it must be regularly inspected and tested to determine that it is operable and effective in an emergency. The Fire Marshal verifies that an adequate water supply is available for firefighters. The Fire Marshal locates, checks, and/or tests the following pieces of fire equipment to confirm they function properly: Control valves; fire pumps; extinguishing systems, including sprinklers and hand-held extinguishers; hydrants; alarms, including both heat and smoke detectors; fire doors; and protective signaling devices. The CHFM designates fire personnel on the maintenance staff or hires a fire contractor. Fire personnel are responsible for replacing deteriorated equipment and low batteries and checking the system. The CHFM orders the copying of fire equipment manuals and arranges for staff fire training. The CHFM keeps a central file of training, manuals, and testing.

AIA

The American Institute of Architects (AIA) was founded in 1857 and is based in Washington, DC. It is the leading professional association for licensed architects in the USA. and Canada. The AIA provides a voice for architects and advocates for the profession. The AIA provides architects with a Code of Ethics and Professional Conduct, and a comprehensive collection of contract documents dealing with the complete range of design and construction for both large and small projects. The AIA also maintains the Architect's Knowledge Resource, which is a collection covering more than 120,000 architectural topics and products. The AIA publishes the mandatory continuing education requirements for architects by state and province. The AIA hosts conferences and events to keep architects current with their market. The Web site for AIA is http://www.aia.org/.

Model Building Codes

Model Building Codes are developed and maintained by standards organizations that do not have jurisdiction over enacting and enforcing the codes but may offer consulting services to the users of the codes. State and local governments may adopt a Model Building Code in its entirety or make minor revisions to it. Some governments adopt only specific portions of the Model Building Codes, usually the electrical, plumbing and fire codes. Using the Model Codes saves a government the time and money that would be required to write their own codes. Among the organizations that have developed Model Codes are the Building Official Code Administrators International, Inc. (BOCA), the International Conference of Building Officials (ICBO), and the Southern Building Code Congress

International, Inc. (SBCCI). The CHFM is responsible for following the codes that pertain to the municipality, county and state in which the facility operates, rather than a model building code.

ADA Requirements

The Americans with Disabilities Act was passed by Congress in 1990. ADA is a federal anti-discrimination statute intended to extend to qualified persons with disabilities the same opportunities for employment and advancement that are available to able-bodied workers. ADA requires that an employer make reasonable accommodations to enable the disabled person to perform the tasks of a job. However, it does not excuse the disabled person from performing those tasks to the same standards that are expected of workers who are not disabled. Accommodations are not standardized for specific positions, but must be tailored by each employer to fit each disabled worker. The CHFM can get assistance with complying with ADA by visiting http://www.ada.gov/ or calling 800-514-0301.

EPA

The Environmental Protection Agency (EPA) is a federal government agency charged with the regulation of chemicals and the protection of human health through the safeguarding of the water, air, and land. The EPA enforces national environmental laws. These two areas of medical waste are major concerns for the EPA:

- Hospital incinerators pollute the air through their flues with heavy metals, carbon monoxide, acid gases, organics, pathogens, and particulates
- Medical facilities pollute water and land by improperly disposing of regulated medical waste (RMW) that could spread diseases, such as hepatitis and HIV from incorrect sharps disposal (used needles, scalpels, lancets, and blades).

The CHFM must follow health regulations by the federal EPA, OSHA, CDC, and DOT, and state regulations. The CHFM can get assistance with pollution prevention and compliance through the Healthcare Environmental Resource Center at http://www.hercenter.org/rmw/rmwoverview.cfm.

Joint Commission

The Joint Commission (formerly the Joint Commission on Accreditation of Healthcare Organizations or JCAHO) is a national not-for-profit organization that accredits and certifies more than 20,000 national and international healthcare programs and organizations through peer reviews. Its mission is to improve patient safety and quality of care. The Joint Commission sets standards for accreditation and competencies for health workers, especially regarding infection control, continuing education, visiting rules, patient rights, background checks, staffing levels, medical records, and ventilation. The Joint Commission issues the National Patient Safety Goals (NPSGs) for outpatient programs and the National Performance Goals (NPGs) for hospital programs annually, under advisement of national experts from the American College of Physicians, the American Hospital Association, and the American College of Surgeons. The Joint Commission requires quality management and risk management be linked. The Joint Commission established core measures to determine if healthcare institutions comply with current standards, and it makes the results of its accreditation surveys public.

NFPA

The National Fire Protection Association (NFPA) is an international, non-profit organization that publishes more than 300 codes and standards to reduce fire risk. NFPA is the leading international advocate for the prevention of fire. The CHFM should subscribe to National Fire Codes Subscription Service to keep current regarding changes in fire, electrical and building safety. NFPA's mission is to reduce "the worldwide burden of fire and other hazards on the quality of life by providing and advocating consensus codes and standards, research, training, and education." NFPA's membership is more than 81,000 persons and trade and professional organizations. The organization impacts the healthcare industry through its codes and standards, especially the Life Safety Code.

OSHA

OSHA is the US Department of Labor's Occupational Safety & Health Administration. OSHA works with the Environmental Protection Agency to develop federal regulations that safeguard the health and safety of American workers. You are required to adopt OSHA regulations as part of your standards of practice. Visit their site at http://www.osha.gov for updates and to download record keeping forms. Keep pertinent regulations in your Quality manual. All hospital and other healthcare employees are affected by OSHA regulations, but particularly housekeepers, groundskeepers, laboratory technicians, Central Sterile Supply and maintenance workers. The CHFM must be familiar with the Bloodborne Pathogens Standard (revised 2001) that protects workers from hepatitis, HIV and other infections spread through contact with bloody aerosols and contaminated sharps. OSHA mandates: Safety devices such as fume hoods and filters; spill clean-up and the Chemical Hygiene Plan; personal protective equipment (PPE); hygiene and grooming; and injury logs.

CDC

The Centers for Disease Control (CDC) in Atlanta are a major component of the US Department of Health and Human Services. The CDC impacts facility management because it develops and provides guidelines to prevent infections among workers in healthcare establishments. The CDC announces outbreaks and provides reliable statistics and tools for investigation. It provides information about emergency preparedness for bioterrorism, mass casualties, chemical and radiation emergencies, natural disasters, severe weather, and food recalls. The CDC encourages safety and provides training in the forms of interactive courses, videos, and publications. Among the healthcare areas of concern to the CDC are: Hand hygiene; the exposure of workers to hazardous drugs, chemicals, waste and communicable diseases; and occupational injuries, such as back injuries, allergies, cuts and needle sticks. To access the CDC's free tools for emergency preparedness, visit http://emergency.cdc.gov/preparedness/.

Building Permits

The general contractor for the project must obtain a building permit before construction can start on a new building or a renovation project involving construction. Building permits are mandated by the local government and depend on compliance with the applicable zoning regulations. Subdivision regulations may also apply. The building permit may reference local codes dealing with electricity, plumbing, HVAC, gas, and the Life Safety Code. The local building inspector must approve the construction documents, which the general contractor has submitted as a complete set, before the local government issues a building permit. Regular inspections of the work occur as the project progresses. The project must comply with all applicable requirements before a certificate of occupancy is issued.

Elevators

The facility manager is responsible for ensuring all elevators and other equipment for moving people and freight are kept in safe operating condition. The facility manager must ensure that routine maintenance and tests are performed by a staff person certified for that duty. If no such person is already on staff, the facility manager must hire someone or contract with an outside agency to perform the service. The facility manager must also ensure that the required operating signage and passenger instructions are posted correctly. Another responsibility of the facility manager is to monitor the operation of the equipment and document his/her observations.

Signage for Elevators and Vertical Transportation Equipment

ASME A17.1-1996 Safety Code for Elevators and Escalators contains a national list of signage for elevators and other vertical transportation equipment. Local governments may not adopt the entire list, but may use only part of it in the local codes. Among the required signs are instructions for what to do in case of fire. Freight elevators must contain statements of capacity and other data including an indication of whether they are freight only or may carry passengers. Dumbwaiters should have signs indicating that they are to be kept closed and that they do not carry passengers. Escalators should have signs that tell passengers to hold the handrail and to attend children. An emergency stop button should also be clearly indicated.

Licensed or Certified Personnel

Licenses or certification are required for several types of facility maintenance work. For example, HVAC workers who handle chlorofluorocarbon-containing refrigerants are required to pass a certification examination approved by the Environmental Protection Agency. The energy management control system should have operators who are trained and certified for their work. Persons working with electrical and HVAC systems should be trained and in many cases must hold a license or certificate. In some situations the work must be contracted to licensed tradesmen, if the company does not employ certified or licensed personnel, such as plumbing, the installation of electrical wiring, and the maintenance of the elevators.

HVAC Technician or Engineer

An HVAC technician or engineer works in the field of heating, ventilation, and air conditioning. He or she can receive certification through a technical school or through participation in an apprenticeship program. A license for personnel who handle or purchase refrigerants is available through an exam administered by the EPA. The duties of the HVAC technician or engineer are likely to include the installation, maintenance, and repair of furnaces, oil burners, air conditioning systems, thermostats, ducts, and vents. Inspections of the heating and air conditioning systems and combustion testing are other duties HVAC workers perform.

Analyzing Indoor Environment

A healthcare establishment must provide a clean, safe environment for its workers, clients, and patients. Much of the indoor environment is determined by the ventilation of the space. State and local codes establish the amount of air that must be circulated through the space. The amount for a particular space may include a quantity of fresh or outdoor air. The amount of ventilation is usually calculated according to the volume of the space or on the square footage. When analyzing the environment, the facility manager must take into consideration the code requirements, the size of the space, the number of occupants, and how the space is used. For example, isolation wards and laboratories have specific OSHA guidelines for reverse pressure airflow and fume hoods. Another important consideration is whether smoking is now allowed in the building or if it has ever been allowed.

Smoke-Free Environments

Smoke-free environments are established in new buildings by never allowing smoking. To create a smoke-free atmosphere in an older building in which tobacco use was previously allowed is a major renovation project because materials in rooms absorb tobacco smoke and continue to emit it back into the air long after smoking in the area has ceased. Smoke is absorbed and emitted by carpet, painted walls, upholstery and other fabrics, drapes and blinds, plastic materials, and absorptive tile ceilings. Cleaning or washing these surfaces is insufficient to make the room or area smoke-free. All absorptive materials must be removed and replaced, except for walls, which must be recovered or carefully washed and repainted.

Factors Reviewed After Fires

Once there has been even a small fire, it is the responsibility of the facility manager to review the event and determine what went wrong and what was done right. First, the facility manager determines if the affected building or the section in which the fire occurred met all applicable codes. The facility manager must then determine if improvements are needed in the fire suppression systems or if the handling procedures for hazardous material or equipment should be changed. The exact cause of the fire is determined by the Fire Marshall and facility manager. The facility manager takes steps to prevent a recurrence. The facility manager ensures that the fire alarm system is adequate and that it functions properly. A review of escape routes may be needed.

Fire Training

The facility manager is responsible for arranging fire training for all staff members and reinforcing it with periodic fire drills. The facility manager designates an in-house fire team or hires a fire contractor. The facility manager establishes evacuation routes with fire personnel and posts maps of the routes in each area of the building. All personnel should know the locations of alarm pull stations and how to activate them. Fire training should also include practice in the use and operation of hand-held extinguishers. Maintenance and Operations personnel must know where specific monitoring panels are located and should have a thorough knowledge of the protocols for shutoff valves and disconnects. The facility manager keeps a permanent log of fire training and supplies the training materials required by instructors.

In-House Fire Response Team

An in-house fire response team is a group of employees trained in the use of fire-fighting equipment. The in-house fire team is able to respond to a fire emergency until the local fire department arrives. A minimum of two persons from each shift is usually included in the in-house fire team. The responsibility for directing the in-house fire team rests with either the Chief Engineer or the Director of Security. The in-house fire team's duties are to: Have hands-on experience with the equipment; be familiar with the locations of all exits, evacuation routes, and procedures; and know how to operate the alarm system. Often, the fire team is also trained in first aid and CPR in case of injury.

In-House Fire Brigade

An in-house fire brigade is a group of employees trained according to OSHA standards to actually fight structural fires. The Safety Officer is the resource for the in-house fire brigade. A fire brigade is needed in medical facilities that are not located near enough to a local volunteer or municipal fire department for quick response. The members of a fire brigade are trained at an approved school for fire fighters and have access to proper personal protective equipment (PPE) and fire-fighting equipment. Since most healthcare facilities are not situated in isolated locations, a fire response team is more likely to be used than a fire brigade. However, isolation hospitals for communicable diseases, Biosafety Level 4 (BSL-4) laboratories, and maximum security hospitals for dangerous offenders may use brigades.

Corrective Action in Fire Protection Systems

Local fire codes are rewritten periodically. The changes to local fire codes are applied retroactively. The CHFM must keep abreast of rewrites to the fire codes, and must replace older equipment and make required changes in the buildings he/she manages. The CHFM may arrange installations, modifications, increases, or updates for:

- Alarms
- Automatic sprinklers
- Door closers
- Elevator emergency controls
- Emergency lighting
- HVAC system
- Maps of evacuation routes and fire safety diagrams
- Smoke controls

When planning for any renovation project, the CHFM must review of local codes thoroughly to determine if any current fire prevention and control measures no longer meet the codes.

Fire Extinguisher Inspection

Designated fire personnel weigh all portable fire extinguishers in the healthcare facility every month to ensure they have not lost any of their chemical content. Wet-chemical extinguishers should undergo a hydrostatic test every 5 years to make sure there is no corrosion or other internal damage. Halon replacement, dry-powder, and dry-chemical extinguishers should undergo the hydrostatic test on a schedule of every 12 years. The designated fire personnel place lead and wire or plastic tamper seals on extinguishers that pass the tests, so that a visual inspection can indicate that there has been no unauthorized use. The facility manager arranges with Emergency Services the annual testing of heliport extinguishers, as the landing pad is closed and medevac patients must be rerouted to another hospital until the test is complete.

Coordination with Community

Fires

Healthcare facilities get a full-tiered response (police, fire department, and ambulance) from EMS in an emergency because:

- Many patients are not ambulatory
- Some patients are confused and may become combative or get lost
- Dangerous chemicals, radiation and infections could be released
- Looting valuable drugs, equipment, and patient files could occur

Nursing and administrative staff focus on evacuating patients, not on saving property. The CHFM ensures:

- Staff are trained to recognize color code announcements (e.g., Code Red for fire)
- Vertical and horizontal evacuation plans are in place for each floor
- Helper locations are notified to receive evacuees
- Community agencies and volunteers are alerted
- Utility companies and vendors are contacted for extra supplies (e.g., portable heaters, incubators, blankets)
- Supply deliveries are stopped or redirected if the facility is closed

The Administrator On-call coordinates public relations and issues statements to the media.

Natural Disasters

When a natural disaster strikes a community, the Multi-Agency Coordination System (MACS) responds. Rescue efforts are conducted by EMS (police, fire department, and ambulance), Red Cross, and military Search and Rescue teams. Healthcare facilities and community agencies, such as Public Health, the CDC, and community care nurses, are second-line responders. Mass casualties require the assistance of private doctors and allied health personnel. Public buildings, such as schools, sports arenas and churches, are used as shelters. Extra medical supplies, food, clean water, and morgues are secured by deputies in case of looting. US states and Canadian provinces follow the Standardized Emergency Management System (SEMS) for natural disaster preparedness, mitigation, response and recovery. The CHFM helps to set up the Incident Command System (ICS) for the healthcare facility. The Administrator On-call liaises with community leaders and designates a spokesperson for the healthcare facility.

Management of Fire Safety Program

The CHFM oversees the healthcare facility's fire safety program, but the program must involve all employees. The fire safety program includes:

- Fire prevention by identifying and removing or controlling hazards
- Maintenance of smoke and fire alarm systems and fire suppression systems (e.g., sprinklers and standpipes)
- Employee training in safe use of necessary hazardous materials and equipment before a fire
- Regular monthly testing of safety equipment
- Developing evacuation plans and posting routes
- Intruder alerts
- Monitoring employee behavior during a fire (caring for patients, safeguarding property, and maintaining confidential patient records)
- Liaison with helper agencies
- Debriefing
- Recovery

Fuel Oil Storage

The facility manager must have a thorough knowledge of the national and local codes concerning the storage and handling of fuel oil. Local codes are likely to control the amount of fuel that is allowed to be stored at the facility, whether it must be stored in above-ground tanks or in tanks underground, and the type and size of piping that must be used to move the fuel from storage to the point where it is burned. In some situations, oil-burning equipment may be located in a basement with the fuel storage also inside. This situation must also meet the safety standards set by the local codes. In most cases, the local codes are based on those established by the National Fire Protection Association (NFPA Code 30, Flammable and Combustible Liquids Code) and the US Department of Transportation (DOT).

Evaluation of Work Performance

Supervisors should inspect and evaluate the work of those they supervise to ensure that any maintenance and repairs do not violate code requirements. Supervision applies to both facility workers and contractors. Regular inspections and feedback are required for proper annual and probationary performance appraisals, pay raises, bonuses, and promotions. The CHFM's review of a worker's performances can also identify needs for remedial training and referral to the Employee Assistance program. The evaluation can be used as the basis for setting individual goals for the next evaluation period. A new hire usually has an evaluation at the end of the probationary period (3 months or 6 months) and annually thereafter. Check the collective agreement or contract of the workers you supervise for the correct timing. Ask a Human Resources officer to accompany you at the performance appraisal, if necessary.

Questionnaires

Questionnaires are used to qualitatively measure requestor satisfaction with response time to work orders by Operations, Maintenance, Engineering, and contractors, and the quality of the work performed. Either ask 10% of all requestors or work-order initiators to randomly complete a questionnaire each month or target a different department to complete a questionnaire in consecutive months. Include the results of the questionnaires in your monthly, quarterly, and annual reports. Custodial services can be measured in the same way, since the cleaning of patient rooms and other public spaces are important for preventing the spread of disease. Custodial services questionnaires can be requested from patients/clients or their caregivers and staff members. Incorporate the results in performance appraisals, if a particular worker or contractor is identified.

Inspection

The facility manager is responsible for daily inspections in these areas, or sending a delegate:

- Food: Preparation surfaces are clean; raw food is stored and handled with proper care; meals are served on time and at the proper temperature.
- Electrical and HVAC: Repairs and maintenance of building systems must be performed by licensed workers to standards set by local codes.
- Housekeeping: The cleanliness of the facility meets the standards of the Infection Control and Quality Assurance teams with regard to cleaning treatment rooms, disposing of clinical waste, and disinfecting common areas.
- Groundskeeping: Law suits are avoided because staff use due diligence when clearing snow, posting warning signs, and securing slippery areas.

Direct observation is the best way to determine that the work is done properly.

Equipment Failure

All equipment fails eventually. In medical settings, even the best equipment has a short lifespan due to the stress of repeated harsh cleaning to remove disease-causing organisms (pathogens) and heavy use by many staff and patients. Defective items fail because of poor workmanship; although the equipment passed reliability testing in the factory, the benchmark was too low. Hospitals have backup generators, but power surges and outages can short circuit machines and cause equipment failure. Other items simply become less effective or efficient as they age, or become obsolete as technology advances. Contaminated equipment that cannot be cleaned is decommissioned. Complicated equipment, such as air conditioners containing many parts, may fail because one particular part is defective or has worn out. Some items are subject to suddenly failure without warning. An example of this is an electric light bulb, which has an average life span, but may fail at any time.

Repair Versus Replacement

The CHFM makes the decision to repair or replace essential building equipment when it fails. Four factors enter into the CHFM's decision:

- Cost of replacement vs. cost of repair — Include the time for in-house personnel to repair the item plus any downtime caused by the item being out of service.
- Contracting out — If the item cannot be repaired in-house, consider the cost of increased downtime of having it repaired by an outside agency, the confidentiality issues, and existing contracts.
- Cascade failure — When a small piece of medical equipment that was bought in bulk fails, inventory other similar items of the same age that may fail in the near future.
- Bulk purchase discounts — Vendors may offer cost discounts for purchasing several of the items likely to fail soon, so it may be cheaper to replace all of them at once, rather than waiting for each to fail sequentially.

Asbestos Abatement

Asbestos is a fibrous mineral that was used before the 1970s as a fire retardant and insulator in building materials. Asbestos needles were usually combined with other materials through the use of strong bonding agents. Bonded asbestos is usually safe. However, when bonded materials become crumbly or damaged, they release fibers into the air that when inhaled cause lung cancer, asbestosis, or mesothelioma. Occupational diseases from asbestos exposure do not appear immediately, but develop many years later. Maintenance activities that can cause a release of fibers from an asbestos-containing material include improper removal, sanding, scraping, cutting and sawing, tearing, and drilling. Gaskets that contain asbestos can release fibers if they become worn. If an inspector determines that a facility has asbestos-containing materials, an abatement program by specially trained workers wearing PPE may be required.

Once an inspector determines that asbestos is present in a building, an abatement program is needed. The most frequent method of eliminating the hazards of asbestos exposure is the removal of all asbestos-containing material under a containment tent and disposing of it as toxic waste. Depending on local codes, some materials may be enclosed or encapsulated. While in-house staff may be trained to abate asbestos, it is usually best to hire a reputable, professional contractor to handle the project. Local codes may require that only certified persons handle the asbestos and dictate the disposal method. The CHFM carefully maintains a record of all asbestos abatement efforts for the EPA, OSHA, and accreditation surveyors.

Mold

Molds are fungi that grow in damp, dark, places below 77°F with humidity above 70%, such as between dividing walls, behind panels and in canals. There are 200,000 harmless species of mold. These species of mold in the USA are harmful to human health: Aspergillus, Alternaria, Stachybotrys (black mold), Cladosporium, Epicoccum, Helminthosporium, Mucor and Penicillium. Water damage in a building encourages mold growth. Mold may or may not produce a scent. Many inhaled mold spores produce mycotoxins, called aflatoxins, trichothecene, beta glucans, and nitric oxides. Mycotoxins cause skin rash, memory loss from brain damage, leukemia, and cancer of the kidney, liver and esophagus. Identify discolored areas indicating water seepage and condensation. Ask your Safety Officer to use a test kit or hire a licensed mold inspector. People with compromised immune systems, allergies, asthma, and sinusitis are most at-risk. Mold targets infants and children, the elderly and pregnant women. Therefore, concentrate your search in respiratory, obstetrics, pediatric, and gerontology wards.

Abatement Program

Some molds are toxic and damage surfaces on which they grow. Prevent mold growth and promote quick cleanup when mold is found. Order leaks and water damage fixed as quickly as possible. If mold is cleaned up, but the underlying moisture problem remains, the mold is likely to return. Areas prone to developing mold include: Air conditioning ducts; humidifiers; vinyl wallpaper over drywall; floor drains; basements; attics; bathrooms; kitchens; mattresses; foam pillows; carpets; upholstery; garbage chutes and containers. Controlling mold means reducing moisture below 55%. Suspect mold if people complain of: Nose or rectal bleeding; headaches; fatigue; memory loss; personality changes; shortness of breath; cough; sore throat; abdominal pain; tremors or numbness; rash; and hair loss. Delegate in-house workers to clean up small moldy areas. They must follow EPA guidelines and wear gloves, goggles, and N-95 respirators. Hire a professional, experienced contractor if the moldy area is large, if there is extensive water damage, or if the HVAC system is contaminated.

Hazardous Waste

Hazardous waste produced by healthcare facilities contains toxic chemicals, radioactive materials, and byproducts of patient testing and treatment. Clinical waste includes:

- Items contaminated with potentially infectious body fluids (urine, feces, saliva, blood, tears, cerebrospinal fluid)
- Sharps (used needles, lancets, and scalpels)
- Body parts
- Expired medications

Sharps require a locked disposal container and must be separated from other items. Building and renovation projects generate other types of hazardous waste, such as asbestos. The disposal of clinical waste and other hazardous materials is controlled by federal law. Some places require that clinical and non-clinical waste be separated so that non-clinical waste can be recycled.

Healthcare organizations utilize four basic approaches to the control of hazardous waste:

- Minimize exposure at the point of waste production — Establish good procedures tailored to the area, especially the Operating Room, Pharmacy, Laboratory, and patient care areas. For example, drug addicts search garbage for needles and medications, so secure Out-patient Clinic garbage.
- Clean and remove — Housekeeping is responsible for checking all areas on a schedule and staff must report spills and contamination as they occur. Clean-up techniques are specific to the risks of the materials involved, and may require specially trained staff with the correct PPE.
- Establish routines according to OSHA's Bloodborne Pathogens Standard — Patients, staff, visitors, EMS personnel, and intruders who were exposed to hazardous waste must all undergo decontamination and prophylaxis or follow-up.
- Epidemiologic study — Whenever the hazardous waste control program fails, alert the Risk Manager, Safety Officer, Infection Control, Security and Public Health, as appropriate to the situation.

It is an insufficient standard of care for the CHFM to simply release hazardous waste to a disposal contractor and think no more about it. The CHFM must either monitor the contractor's performance and safety record personally, or hire an environmental hygienist to monitor in-house collection and the contractor's procedures for handling, storing, and disposing of the hazardous materials. Both federal and local codes may apply to the disposal of various types of hazardous waste. Seek competent legal advice regarding the specific types of waste your facility produces. Your Risk Manager, Infection Control and Safety Officer can help you. Any waste management contractor your facility hires should have a good reputation and be experienced. It is fair to ask for references, licenses or certificates, and to order a background check.

Life Safety Code

NFPA 101: Life Safety Code is a document published by the National Fire Protection Association. NFPA 101 is a consensus standard and becomes a legal code only when it is adopted by a state or local authority. The Life Safety Code sets standards for both existing buildings and new construction. According to the NFPA Website, the Life Safety Code is concerned with "those construction, protection, and occupancy features necessary to minimize danger to life from fire, heat, and toxic gasses created during a fire." The Code also sets minimum standards for exits, in order to allow occupants to escape promptly from buildings. Other items covered by the Life Safety Code include maintenance activities, protective systems, and operating features.

Safety Program Elements

Your safety program must comply with OSHA, which sets detailed standards for safety and health. OSHA also requires specific recordkeeping by employers. Among the elements that you must include in your safety program is limited access to work areas. Strictly control access to: Roofs; helipads; tools; chemicals; laboratories; drug cupboards; morgues; research, electrical, HVAC, and telephone rooms. Post warnings of danger in appropriate areas. Encourage staff to take care not to create unnecessary hazards by placing wires or hoses in traffic paths. Work areas should be cleaned promptly. OSHA offers a free online tool to help you design your safety program correctly, at: http://www.osha.gov/SLTC/etools/hospital/index.html.

Coordination of Departments During Disasters

All local hospitals will be involved when a disaster strikes a community, no matter if it is a natural disaster, such as a hurricane, or something manmade, such as a dirty bomb. Emergency Preparedness plans are made ahead according to the Standardized Emergency Management System (SEMS). Each administrator and department head knows exactly what he or she is expected to do in SEMS, and where the Incident Command Center will be. The CHFM works with Human Resources to obtain additional personnel, which may involve contacting retirees. The CHFM oversees the rearrangement of space to accommodate a triage area and the larger number of patients. The CHFM must understand work refusal and work stoppage policies and procedures. Duties are shifted or rearranged so that the care of current patients will not be interrupted by the influx of disaster victims. The CHFM liaises with Engineering and Operations to make arrangements for backup utilities.

Safety Committees

Every healthcare organization must establish its own Patient Safety Committee, charged with maintaining safe delivery of patient care. The CHFM is directly connected with the Patient Safety Committee because of the Housekeeping and Maintenance functions involved in patient care. Another type of safety committee is more concerned with the physical environment of the building and grounds, especially the reduction and elimination of fire hazards and the causes of accidents. The CHFM works closely with the latter committee to deal with incidents or with potential problems as they are identified. The CHFM deals with the Safety Officer, a full-time safety coordinator with no competing duties. The Safety Officer ranks highly within the organization and has authority to make safety decisions and change processes. The Safety Officer helps the CHFM to:

- Arrange for staff training and inspections
- Organize safety teams
- Assess risk
- Measure performance
- Contact external agencies and internal stakeholders
- Write policies and procedures
- Maintain the error reporting system

Security Service

The Security Service of a healthcare facility provides protection for employees, clients/ patients, and the property. Security officers investigate threats of violence and acts of theft and vandalism. Security officers monitor property open to damage and looting, such as during a natural disaster. Security is also concerned with traffic control, access control, identification of personnel, and the creation of an environment that is reassuring to persons with a legitimate reason for being at your facility. Security officers discourage disruptive, violent, or destructive behavior. The Security Service employs uniformed guards who are either in-house employees or from a contracted service. The healthcare Security Service works closely with local fire and law enforcement organizations.

Security System Elements

A good security system is composed of three basic elements:

- Personnel — Security officers are usually uniformed so they are easily recognizable, but occasionally they are undercover. Security officers are responsible for enforcing the hospital's Policies & Procedures. They deal with problems, including alarms, and investigate accidents and incidents.
- Devices — Devices include: Both indoor and outdoor lighting; alarms of various types; emergency call boxes in common areas such as parking lots; and locked doors to restricted areas.
- Policies & Procedures (P&P) — P&Ps establish the limits for access and movement at the hospital. P&Ps detail the proper response to particular situations in the correct sequence (algorithm), including identifying and reporting problems. A guideline is only a recommendation, and does not have the same force as a P&P.

Joint Commission's Statement of Conditions

Every accredited healthcare facility must comply with The Joint Commission's Electronic Statement of Conditions (eSOC) as of September 2007. The CHFM completes the eSOC questionnaire online. According to the introduction and instructions portion of the Statement of Conditions document, the "SOC compliance document has been developed to help you create and maintain a fire safe environment of care and demonstrate compliance with the intent of standards that require newly constructed and existing environments of care be designed and maintained to comply with the Life Safety Code".

The Statement of Conditions document has four parts:

- Part 1 is the Introduction and Instructions
- Part 2 is Basic Building Information

- Part 3 is Life Safety Assessment
- Part 4 is Plan for Improvement

Maintenance and Repair of Medical Equipment

The goal of the equipment repair program should be preventive rather than the fixing of broken items. The CHFM works with Medical Engineering, Operations, the Safety Officer, Quality Assurance Manager, the Heliport Manager, and Maintenance to schedule routine inspections and equipment service. The CHFM keeps a log of all servicing and the replacement of parts. Items should be withdrawn from service and repaired or replaced before they actually break. If there is no Medical Engineering Department, staff members in each department may be trained in the repair of clinical equipment, but it is likely that such items will be sent to an outside repair service. Large items that cannot be moved easily, such as an MRI machine, may be serviced or repaired in place by a contracted vendor.

Management of Utilities Systems Equipment

While utilities for outpatient healthcare establishments differ little from other commercial operations, hospitals and other inpatient organizations have specialized needs. The utility systems must deliver air, water, and steam at differing temperatures and pressures. Critical areas like the Operating Room and Intensive Care Unit must have an uninterrupted power supply. A licensed boiler operator is required for the higher levels of steam pressure. Isolation rooms require filtered air and piped-in oxygen and suction. Ideally, electric power should be supplied from at least two separate substations, with emergency backup power available from on-site generating equipment. It is vital that the equipment for these utilities be properly maintained, repaired, and replaced as needed. The CHFM oversees a continuous supply of utilities and notifies staff when testing will occur.

Hazard Survey

A hazard survey is part of the Safety Committee's work. The hazard survey involves a walk-through inspection of a particular part of a facility or of the entire facility. Usually, the Risk Manager, Infection Control Nurse, Quality Assurance Manager and Safety Officer are included in the walk-through. Representatives from Maintenance and Operations provide keys and lead the committee members through unfamiliar territory. During the survey, Safety Committee members observe and ask questions. They make note of items and situations that pose a danger to personnel, patients, or visitors. Noted hazards range from items out-of-place that could cause someone to trip or that block a passage to something that is a fire hazard. The department supervisor follows up immediately to correct hazards located by the survey team and reports back to the Safety Committee.

Deferred Maintenance

Deferred maintenance means repairs and cleaning that are put off until a later date. Such a delay may be necessitated by budget restraints, timing, or the temporary unavailability of a part, but should not occur because of negligence. Deferred maintenance should not be allowed to become non-maintenance, and care must be taken to ensure that the delayed maintenance does not become a hazard to health, safety, security, or the environment. The deferred item should remain on the maintenance schedule, so that it is not forgotten and management is aware that it has not yet been serviced. Accreditation surveyors inquire about deferred maintenance. If an item is not compliant, then it may result in preliminary denial of accreditation. The CHFM has 90 days following the survey to successfully address all requirements for improvement.

Drills

Hospitals ascribe to emergency color codes, but the system in the USA is not yet standardized. For example, Code Red is mostly announced for fire, but fire can also be "Paging Dr. Firestone", "Dr. Pyro", or "Dr. Red", depending on the hospital's location and if it is a civilian or military facility. Hospital staff rehearse their responses to emergency codes through regularly scheduled drills. Fire drills are rehearsed monthly under the Safety Officer's directions because fire is an ever-present threat. Various types of emergencies and disasters are covered by drills: Lockdown; violent attacks; severe weather; bomb threats; child abduction; chemical spills; escaped patient; and mass casualties. The color code system is part of Orientation training for all personnel, so each employee is aware of how he or she should behave during a crisis. Elaborate mock disasters are drills used for training EMS personnel (fire, police, and ambulance) at the hospital, usually on an annual basis.

Planning, Design & Construction

ICRA

Infection Control Risk Assessment (ICRA of 2006) is a multidisciplinary and organization-wide inspection to reduce infection risks. The in-house Infection Control Manager may lead the ICRA team or the facility may hire an independent contractor. The ICRA inspectors consider both the programs the facility offers and the patient population it serves. The phases of the ICRA are: Planning; design; construction; renovation; and maintenance. The elements of the ICRA are processes for design, construction and mitigation.

- Design involves planning isolation rooms with air filters, vents, fume hoods, water systems, and surfaces that reduce or control the threat of pathogens
- Construction involves limiting disruptions caused by power outages, debris clean-up, and testing for certification by rerouting traffic
- Mitigation involves relocating susceptible patients to protected areas, erecting dust and noise barriers, and training staff.

ILSM

The Interim Life Safety Measures (ILSM) is a guide to mitigate hazards caused by construction. It was developed by The Joint Commission to protect the health and safety of patients, staff, and visitors. The ILSM also compensates for deficiencies in the Life Safety Code. ILSM recommends 36 mitigation measures, including:

- Way-finding helps, such as exit signs and marked pathways
- Fire protection items, such as alarms, fire extinguishers, fire suppression systems and smoke barriers
- Hand railings
- Power tools and cords properly grounded and operational
- Hard hats
- Capped exhaust ducts

The US military publishes an excellent ILSM daily checklist form for the project manager at: http://www.usace.army.mil/CEMP/MX/Documents/ilsm-icra.pdf.

Feasibility Studies

A feasibility study is an engineering evaluation that is part of the planning for a renovation or new construction. The CHFM assembles quantitative data to illustrate the practicability of a particular course of action. The CHFM prepares one study for each possible solution to the problem. Feasibility studies are used to determine the recommended solution. The feasibility study should include information on estimated costs, including any real estate purchase, construction, installation, and the price of new equipment. The feasibility study should also address the proposed facility configuration, any loss of production time, and the costs to relocate personnel, equipment, and systems. List sources (vendors), materials prices, and the availability of transportation, communications, energy, and utilities.

Construction Cost Estimate Items

A construction cost estimate should include costs for site development, construction, operating, support equipment, and a miscellaneous category for design, inspections, and relocation costs. Site-development costs include: Clearing and grading a new site; paving access roads, walks, and parking lots; installing utilities (electricity, water, and sewerage); erecting fencing and lighting; and landscaping. Construction costs include everything that goes into actually building the new facility or the renovation, including materials and building systems. Operating costs are the costs to maintain and repair the facility, including custodial services, security, fire protection, and insurance. Support equipment costs include furnishings, installed equipment, and equipment for the maintenance shop.

Design Firm Selection

The CHFM may be directly assigned to hire an outside design firm by the hospital's administrators. However, some medical facilities use a committee of in-house experts to make the selection through a Request for Proposal. The Selection Committee members might include:

- Persons with expertise in design, life and safety, telecommunications and networking
- Delegates from Engineering, Purchasing, and Building Operations

But whatever the makeup of the Committee, the selection should be controlled by the facility manager. The selected design firm should be able to offer verifiable experience and technical knowledge and should demonstrate cooperativeness. The firm should not be chosen on the basis of its creativity and awards.

Design Team

Small construction projects might be handled successfully by your current staff, but a major project often involves the work of specialists, such as an architect or interior designer, who are not part of your facility's staff. Even when the needed specialists or other personnel are already onboard, they usually have regular duties that would preclude their having the time needed to work on a major project. Large projects usually require contract staff who can devote full time exclusively to the new work. Contractors commonly include: A project manager; an accountant; an engineer; a contracting officer; an architect, and an interior designer.

Build Versus Renovate

Several factors enter into the decision to build a new facility, rather than renovate the current one:

- The organization should determine whether renovation would be mostly cosmetic or if functional changes are needed. If functional changes are necessary, the extent of alterations must be addressed.
- The age of the facility must be considered, along with any changes that would be required because of the Hill-Burton Act of 1947, the updating of the National Electrical Code in 1967, and the identification of asbestos as an environmental hazard in 1972.
- The impact of renovation on the code status of the facility, the levels of usage and the impact of changing technology, and the disruption to the operation of the facility that renovation will cause must be considered.

Contract Negotiation

Construction contracts are often awarded through a sealed-bid process. Another method of procurement for both professional and technical services is the negotiated contract. The negotiation process starts when the hospital administration publishes a Request for Proposals (RFP). The RFP should establish what is to be done and the qualifying criteria, such as experience and specialized personnel. An RFP is the method usually used when the work will cost more than $25,000 and the decision about which company to hire cannot be based solely on the lowest price.

Negotiated contracts allow discussion and flexibility with the possibility of a modification of requirements or offers. The resulting proposals should be evaluated carefully by the Selection Committee, according to technical and financial criteria that have been determined before the proposals are received.

Contract Administration

Contract administration is a function of the CHFM that is technical rather than legal. The CHFM carefully monitors the work of the contractor to ensure that it meets the terms of the contract. The CHFM reports the contractor's failures to meet the contract terms to the medical facility's Legal Department. Contract administration means the CHFM is responsible for the following duties:

- Bidding or contract negotiation
- Evaluating bids or price offers
- Selecting a contractor (sometimes as leader of the Selection Committee)
- Handling change orders
- Authorizing paperwork necessary for payment
- Supervising inspections
- Handling claims
- Contract close-out

The Office of Federal Procurement Policy (OFPP) publishes A Guide to Best Practice for Contract Administration at http://www.acquisition.gov/bestpractices/bestpcont.html.

Design Review

Establish a formal procedure for reviewing the design drawings early in your project. Most CHFMs use automated design review software, such as Autodesk. Include the feasibility study and any concept drawings produced by a design firm in your review. Compare the design to the requirement specifications.

- The first design review should be at the 25% or 35% completion point, when substantial changes can still be made
- Conduct another review at the 80% to 85% completion point, to allow finishing touches to be added
- Conduct a final review when the design is 100% complete but before actual work starts on the building or renovation.

Builder Selection

Choose builders carefully, whether you need them for renovation projects or new construction:

- Interview several builders who have worked before in your local community, so you can see their completed projects.
- Personally interview the manager of each company the builder uses as a reference to overcome the frequent lack of any real information in a reference.
- Select the builder who has completed a number of successful projects that are similar to the one your facility is planning.
- Ask the builder you are considering to demonstrate his firm's financial stability so you know work will probably not be halted due to bankruptcy.
- Meet the proposed project manager to determine if he/she is qualified and compatible with staff at your facility.
- Base your evaluation on common sense rather than bureaucratic procedures.

Gross and Net Square Footage

Gross space or gross square footage refers to the "footprint" of an area and includes walls, partitions, internal corridors, minor utility columns and the usable spaces. Net space or net square footage refers to the space within an area, department, or room that is actually usable. Net square footage can be defined as the area inside the walls of a space or room. Department gross square feet is the designation most often used in facility planning. Department gross square feet is the "footprint" for a particular department, but does not include such common areas as lobbies, public corridors, elevators, stairwells, toilet facilities, exterior walls, major mechanical spaces, and such shared spaces as housekeeping storage.

Construction Contracts

A guaranteed maximum price contract fixes a maximum cost for the project and encourages the contractor to bring the project to completion at a lower cost.

- A cost plus percentage contract allows a fixed percentage to cover overhead and profit for the contractor. This type of contract does not encourage the contractor to cut costs.
- A cost plus fixed fee contract limits the cost ceiling and sets the profit margin.
- A cost plus fixed fee with upset figure contract fixes a cost ceiling while allowing the contractor to make a profit if the costs are lower than the ceiling.

Construction Schedules

Develop a timetable or schedule before the actual start of construction. Most CHFMs use construction scheduling software, such as Microsoft Project, BuildIT, or VirtualBoss, because the entire project may require more than a year. Include the start date and expected finish date for the construction of the project in the schedule. Indicate the expected completion dates for several major divisions or phases of the project. Make your schedule flexible, since problems may be caused by weather, materials availability, labor issues, and other disruptions. It is the responsibility of the facility manager to monitor the schedule and ensure that each phase of the work is completed on time. Software reminders make it easier to monitor the completion of each major task.

Partnering

The details of partnering vary from one project to another, but it is a structured process through which the partners encourage innovation, teamwork and problem solving by the team, and Continuous Quality Improvement (CQA). Typical characteristics of a partnering agreement include: A clear role for each partner; the establishment of common goals and objectives; the establishment of project priorities; a commitment to the sharing of information; a method for sharing information and lessons learned; training; methods of building trust and resolving differences; and the establishment of methods for measuring success.

Design Plans

These five plans are each of a specific floor of a building:

- The base plan is a drawing on which permanent and structural features are indicated.
- A demolition plan is a drawing on which walls or partitions, electrical units, plumbing, telephones, and such features as cabinets and other built-ins that are to be removed are indicated. Demolition plans are used in renovations and remodeling projects only.
- The installation plan indicates the locations of modular panels and the sources and locations for electrical power.

- The component plan indicates the locations of components to be placed on the panels and specific lighting for workstations.
- The floor plan indicates the placement of furniture.

Renderings and Perspectives

Renderings and perspectives are design drawings that present a three-dimensional (3D) view of an enclosed space rather than providing instructions to a builder or installer. Most CHFMs and designers use AutoCAD software for 3D drawings. The drawings may not be to scale. They show the space as it will be seen by a user, and include the colors and textures that are to be used. Furniture and the relationship of the furnishings to the architectural features of the space are represented in the drawings. Renderings, which cost more than scaled drawings, can be used to show administrators and other users how the finished space will look.

Reviewing Shop Drawings

Shop drawings are drawings that a contractor produces to show what and how he expects to build to meet the terms of his contract. The CHFM reviews the drawings to determine that the contractor is staying within the parameters of the design for the project, because the end product is the responsibility of the CHFM. The CHFM gives the contractor clear guidelines for the project. The contractor may need to produce only one set of shop drawings. However, if the contractor is hired before the final determination of the scope or design of the project is established, then he/she makes a set of drawings for each possibility. It is the CHFM's responsibility to provide adequate guidance to the contractor and to review the drawings.

Baseline Data for Planning

Baseline data must be compiled at or before the start of the planning process. Include the following internal baseline data in your planning: Range of current services; patient mix; number of staff; scheduling patterns and workloads; major diagnostic and treatment units; the age and continuing life expectancy of the equipment; floor plans of the departments; and the numbers of inpatient beds and nursing stations. The collected data should also include an external site plan with boundaries indicated, traffic patterns, parking, and entrances to all buildings. Expected changes in services, patient mix, and technology should be part of the data. Current deficiencies should also be indicated.

Predesign Planning

Predesign planning should be the first stage of a construction or renovation project. The CHFM makes a set of decisions to guide the project through its design, construction and operations. During redesign planning, the CHFM puts into words and conceptual drawings general concepts of what is needed. The CHFM determines how this project fits into the organization's strategic and business plans. The CHFM establishes size of the project, including square footage, staffing, and new equipment, along with the expected effects of technology. The CHFM identifies the exact location and states whether the project is to be a new facility or renovation of the current one. The CHFM uses a sensitivity analysis to determine if the project is feasible by estimating the costs and revenues for internal rates of return (IRR).

Lack of Preplanning

It is a mistake for the CHFM to rushing into the design phase of a building or renovation project before completing predesign planning. Lack of predesign planning can result in a facility that is overbuilt or not entirely appropriate for its purpose. An incompletely designed project does not fit well into the organization's overall strategy for capital investment and may cause an unjustified increase in operating costs. Predesign planning can be used to produce a facility that fits the needs of the current organization and that has the flexibility and adaptability to meet changes in technology and medical practice in the future.

Project Quality Control

Quality control of a project involves inspection by the architect of the project, but may become more the responsibility of in-house personnel. Quality control requires:

- Careful selection of contractors for the project. Efforts to screen out those who do not have a satisfactory record will result in more reliable and capable workers.
- Frequent review and oversight by the facility manager and the Experts Committee to ensure that the project is completed on time, within budget, according to design, and that all applicable code requirements are met.
- Hiring a construction inspector for a large project, who is qualified for the type of construction that is underway.

Benchmarks

Benchmarks are points of reference or standards against which something can be measured or judged. Healthcare benchmarks are measured by surveyors for facility accreditation. Benchmark types useful in facilities planning include the ability of the physical plant to carry the current workload, the overall adequacy of departmental spaces provided for procedure areas, the productivity of the spaces, and the efficiency of the spaces, which may be a net-to-gross ratio. Spaces are commonly measured in department gross square feet (DGSF). Benchmarks can be used in the development of preliminary estimates of space needs in a new or renovated facility.

Questions Regarding Upgrading or Expansion

Before making the decision to spend the funds to upgrade or expand a department, the CHFM must ask the following six questions and determine credible, accurate answers:

- Could changes such as expanding the hours of operation or reconfiguring the department eliminate the need to upgrade?
- Could the department be moved to a location that would facilitate the sharing of staff or procedure rooms with another department?
- Would the relocation enhance client and patient service?
- What is the current age and condition of the equipment involved?
- Is it up-to-date or is new equipment needed?
- Are current support spaces adequate to meet the needs of staff and patients?

Change Order

A change order is a written form by which a company can alter the Scope of Work section of the contract with a builder or other contractor. The project manager costs the change and generates the order. Many change orders can be made over the course of a large project. Change orders solve problems with incorrect estimates, substitutes, construction obstacles, budget changes, and demands for new features. They can be used to alter the quantity of what is provided or the quality or method of the work. Change orders can also be used to modify details of the design. Once the facility and the contractor have agreed on the requested change, the change order becomes a legal contract.

Request for Information

A request for information (RFI) is a common business practice in which a business collects information about potential suppliers to make a supply or service decision. The collected information is in written form, and the RFI is usually constructed in a table or grid so the information from various companies can be compared. Requests for information are often used in conjunction with or in preparation for a request for proposal, a request for quotation, or a request for tender. In construction, a RFI can be used to confirm a detail or specification. It is also acceptable for a subcontractor or vendor to use an RFI to express concern about inferior products or the misuse of a product, or to clarify the intended use of a product by the owner of the building.

Status Reports to Management

The CHFM makes regular reports on the status of a project to the Policy Committee and the CEO of the healthcare facility throughout the duration of a project. It is a good idea to also share the reports with the senior user of the new or renovated facility and the supervisor to whom the CHFM reports. The CHFM should present a progress report in person, in case the CEO and Committee members have questions. The CHFM should be fully-informed and well-rehearsed before giving the report. Use several forms of media, including printed handouts, video, and slide show presentations. When the project involves ideas or technology that are new or innovative, mockups may be helpful. Mockups can sometimes be supplied by a vendor.

Policy Committee

A Policy Committee is the top level of direction and control for a major project. The lower level Experts Committee has less authority and responsibility. The Committee is chaired by a high-level executive, such as a vice-president. Members of the Committee include a representative from the Controller's office, legal counsel, the facility manager, the project manager, and the manager of the design or construction team. The Committee is responsible for approving any major changes in the project, keeping the CEO and Board of Directors informed of progress and problems, and dealing with issues forwarded to it from the Experts Committee. The Chair sends out the agenda prior to an upcoming meeting, and the Secretary keeps Minutes as a legal obligation.

Preparation and Follow-Up for Meetings

The Chair prepares an agenda and the Secretary distributes it at least 24 hours before the meeting. The agenda should include an update on the progress of the project, a comparison of current expenditures to the projected budget, and a statement of whether or not the project is progressing on time. The Secretary accepts regrets and keeps a list of attendees. The meeting may be cancelled by the Chair if there is no quorum (not enough people to vote on a decision). The Chair asks the members to accept the Minutes of the last meeting. The Chair allows time for the discussion of old business, new business, and any new problems that have arisen. The Chair may review who is doing what. Each Committee member provides a progress report. No more than 48 hours after the meeting, the Secretary follows up by circulating the Minutes. An additional 48 hours should be sufficient for any amendments to the Minutes.

Experts Committee

An Experts Committee is the lower of two levels of direction and control for a major project. The higher level Policy Committee has more authority and responsibility. A typical Experts Committee is made up of the: Project Manager; design team manager; the builder's manager; in-house design chief, Operations chief, Engineering chief; legal counsel; project accountant; the chief inspector; a Security or safety representative; and a staff representative. The Experts Committee is responsible for making the daily decisions that allow the project to progress on schedule and within the budget. The Experts Committee refers issues to the Policy Committee.

Post-Occupancy Evaluation

The facility's administration orders a post-occupancy evaluation approximately six to 18 months after a major project is completed and the new or renovated facility is occupied. The evaluation may be performed by in-house personnel or a hired consulting firm that specializes in post-occupancy evaluations. The post-occupancy evaluation should measure how well the goals of the project program were met. The process should also include gathering information from the staff and users of the facility (patients, visitors, and family members) concerning the program's effects. The CHFM may solicit opinions from special interest groups, such as Emergency Medical Technicians, police, or disabled people who frequent the new area. Needed corrections and adjustments should be identified, along with any corrective action that should be taken for any similar project in the future.

Punch List

A punch list is a list of tasks that must be accomplished – put simply, it is a "to do" list. In the American construction industry, a punch list is a contract document that is used when completing a project. It is a list of items identified during an inspection of the substantially-completed project as incomplete or failing to meet the specifications of the contract. Punch list items might be equipment or material that is not installed correctly, non-functioning equipment, a portion of the project that has not been completed, or un-repaired damage. Final payment for the project is made after all the items on the punch list have been completed or corrected.

As-Built Drawings and Operational Tests

As-built drawings are construction drawings that are modified from their original form in order to show changes made during the building process. They may be derived from prints that have been marked with the changes, other drawings, and additional information supplied by the contractor.

Operational tests determine whether a building's mechanical and electrical equipment and systems are functioning properly. The tests are devised by the company that owns the building and may be used as part of a check on quality before a project is accepted as completed.

Turnover of Project from Builder to Owner

When a major project is completed, there are several procedures that should be involved in the turnover from the builder to the owner:

- Punch lists should be completed
- Operating tests of all equipment and building systems should be completed by the hired inspector and owner's staff
- Any necessary training for the staff should be conducted
- Documentation should be given to the owners, to include: As-built drawings; warranties; schematics and instruction books for equipment; and maintenance information for equipment

A best practice called commissioning may be used to handle the turnover. According to The Facility Management Handbook by David G. Cotts, "Commissioning is the effective and efficient turnover of a major project or building from the builder to the owner and occupants."

Work Handled as Projects

Routine work and preventative maintenance should not be turned into projects. Project status may be based on dollar value (above a specified amount, such as $5,000) or the amount of planning and design required. Capital projects usually involve renovation, modification, or new construction, but likely would not involve the purchase of new furniture or furnishings, unless they were part of a new or renovated facility. Annual projects that are discretionary or that are not too urgent to be delayed, non-routine services, work requiring a high level of user involvement, and major repairs should be handled as projects.

Capital and Churn Projects

Capital projects are large projects that are financed with capital funds rather than through the facility's Operations budget. Capital projects must be approved by an upper level administrator because they are strategic operations, and require large amounts of time and money. Capital projects may involve real estate acquisition and major construction. Churn projects are less expensive than capital projects. Churn projects require less preparation and are often paid for from a departmental budget. Churn projects may involve the relocation of employees and may be for the purpose of changing the function of an area. Some construction and/or renovation may be part of the project.

Upgrading Building Systems

Building systems, such as the HVAC and electrical, should be checked periodically to ensure that they are performing as expected and that they continue to meet the requirements of the facility. Building systems checks should identify equipment that is not operating at optimum efficiency or that is developing problems, such as overheating or excessive vibration. The severity of the inefficiency or operating problem determines whether the equipment should be repaired, replaced, or moved to an area where it will get only light use. Electrical and communication systems may need enhancement or replacement when they are no longer sufficient to meet current needs.

Software for Program Management

The United States Department of Defense has been one organization active in the development of sophisticated project management systems. Computers have enabled the automation of such systems, and software has been developed for both mainframe and personal computers. Microsoft Project is one example of commercially available software for automating project management. It is a management tool that makes functions available to a facility manager that once could be used solely by firms specializing in project management. Some project management software systems have the ability to manage multiple small projects.

Outpatient Services

Renovation or new construction can consolidate various Outpatient, Pre-Admission, and Same-Day testing, treatments and procedures that were scattered throughout the facility. Patients are less stressed by "one-stop shopping". Same-Day services include such procedures as endoscopies, IV therapy, blood transfusions, biopsies, and imaging procedures. Scattered procedure units may have redundant areas for check-in, waiting, preparation, and recovery that could be combined into a shared area as part of a medical procedure unit. A medical procedure unit needs a reception area, change rooms with lockers, a family waiting area, preparation spaces, procedure spaces or rooms to accommodate the services offered by the unit, a recovery room with resuscitation area, and the necessary support space.

ICU Alternatives

Some hospitals consider alternatives to traditional Intensive Care Units as a way of dealing with economic and staffing problems. Patients in traditional ICUs require one-on-one nursing care and are prone to dangerous antibiotic-resistant infections because of the high humidity, warmth, and low lighting. Patient rooms that are acuity-adaptable allow critically ill patients to be monitored and cared for without the need for placement in a special unit. Cardiac patients recovering from invasive procedures can be monitored for 12 to 24 hours in a Day Recovery Center rather than in a Cardiac ICU. Patients who are dependent on ventilators can be cared for in a Chronic Ventilator Unit. Patients with chest pain can be observed and evaluated in a Chest Pain Center rather than being admitted to a Cardiac ICU.

Operational and Space Program Document

The Operational and Space Program document provides all the information needed by the design architect when he or she begins the schematic design for a project. The OSP document should be developed through the process of examining and rethinking: operational processes; technology use; the enhancement of operational efficiency; facility investments; compliance with the applicable codes; aesthetic considerations; and improvements in services to clients and patients. Once approved by the administration, the document can function as a control mechanism for the members of the design team during the development of the design for the project.

Bedside Computing

Bedside computing is a real-time computing system that links all patient care activities, including prescriptions, lab tests, nursing protocols, and charting procedures. Some systems also accept information from telemetry devices that monitor the vital signs of a patient. Bedside computing systems can significantly reduce the amount of time caregivers must spend on paperwork, such as charting. Accounting can use the procedure codes for billing purposes. Bedside systems reduce medication and charting mistakes. Bedside computing allows the real-time sharing of patient data among all personnel involved in the care of that patient, including consultants who are off-site. Bedside computing makes tracing easier for Quality Assurance, Risk Management and Infection Control staff.

System Requirements

Here are the features of an effective bedside computing system:

- Ease of use
- Sharp displays and graphics
- Fast processor
- Sufficient power and memory for the workload
- In-room equipment is small, durable, and well-insulated to withstand accidents such as being dropped, or knocked over, or sprayed with chemicals or body fluids
- Flexibility and expandability to grow with the organization
- Customizable software
- Able to network with all other organization computers, so that data can be quickly and easily shared throughout the organization
- Does not add significantly to the capital costs on a per-bed basis
- Strong back-up and security that meets HIPAA standards

Telecommunications Planning

Telephone lines and the newer fiber optic systems are used increasingly for sending and receiving faxes, videotexts, and other types of data transfer. The infrastructure of the facility must support networking for the organization's computer system and both in-house and outside telephone calls. Lines must be secure to comply with privacy laws (HIPAA). When the CHFM plans for a new structure or a renovation, he/she must include locations for risers, frame rooms, servers, cabinets and closets, fiber-optic runs, cable trays, outlets, antennas, and outside service entry points. Since many architectural-engineering firms do not have the expertise to design the needed system for data transfer and telecommunications, the CHFM must often contract the services of a communications specialist.

Socially Responsible Design

There are five characteristics of socially responsible design:

- The design is based on a value system that is shared by patients, staff, and visitors.
- The design is based on information gathered through interviews and surveys of users, a literature review, visits to other facilities, and the development of potential designs through the use of simulations.
- The design is developed through a participatory process that helps to mesh the objectives of the users and planners with those of the architects and designers.
- Regular, systematic review of the design is part of the process.
- Periodic evaluation of the completed project is an ongoing process.

Design Flexibility

Design flexibility is becoming increasingly important for healthcare facilities to be cost-effective. Three factors contribute to the need for flexibility:

- Changes in the population served by the facility, such as increased ethnics
- Changing needs of the patient population that necessitate alterations in services or service delivery, such as increased elders
- New technology requirements for different spaces and infrastructure amendments

Diagnostic equipment is much larger now than the equipment in use only a few years ago. An example is an MRI machine, which are becoming more popular than the smaller and cheaper x-ray machines. Such size increases may continue, or nanotechnology and other electronic subminiaturization may make large diagnostic equipment obsolete and reduce the space required. Healthcare facilities need to be able to expand or decrease spaces as needed.

Base Construction Cost vs. Total Project Cost

The base construction cost of a renovation project can be estimated as a percentage of the cost of new construction depending on whether the renovation is minor, moderate or major. Once the CHFM estimates the base construction cost, the total project cost can be estimated by adding the anticipated costs for: Site work; parking; the movable equipment to be included; furniture and other furnishings; fees for consultants, architects, interior designers, etc.; the cost of any land acquired; fees for testing and inspections; and financing costs. The CHFM should add a contingency factor of 10% to cover costs that cannot be identified at the beginning of the project.

Request for Bids

The facility manager must assemble a list of exact requirements before publishing a Request for Bids. The list of requirements applies for construction, professional services, or any other work. The CHFM's list of written requirements provides potential bidders with: The project specifications; the exact requirements for the job; price level; certification of personnel who will do specialized work; specific materials to be used; and maintenance that will be required. The Request for Bids may also indicate that the bidder must supply references and examples of previous projects to qualify for consideration. Government facilities usually post RFBs on their Web sites. Private facilities may publish RFBs in the local newspaper or send a mailing to local contractors.

Information Technology Changes

The growth of the Internet and the development of smaller, faster, and more powerful computers have led to many changes in various areas of healthcare. It is no longer necessary for a specialist to be present in a hospital or other healthcare facility in order to consult and exchange information with local doctors. Doctors, nurses, and other healthcare workers can input information from tests and examinations into laptops from which the data can be immediately shared with all personnel concerned with the case. Records for facility, financial, and administrative functions can be fully integrated, leading to better and timelier maintenance and repair. Planning for a new facility or for a renovation must take into consideration the current state of the organization's use of Information Technology and likely updates and expansions. The CHFM should consult with the IT manager as part of preplanning.

Interstitial Spaces

Interstitial spaces are service floors built between the primary floors of a structure. Interstitial spaces provide safe, secure room for electrical, HVAC, and other mechanical services without creating obstructions or hazards on the primary floors. The interstitial floors are usually 6 ft. to 8 ft. high. They allow access for maintenance, repairs, upgrading, and major changes to the building systems without interfering with the offices, treatment areas, and patient rooms on the primary floors. The flexibility interstitial spaces provide can be very important to a healthcare facility, but the cost they add to a building put them beyond the budget of many organizations.

Working with Contractors

Over the past several years, design firms and other businesses have become much more accepting of the facility manager as their chief contact representing the healthcare organization. The facility manager often has the responsibility of communicating all the requirements and needs of his organization to the firms involved in a project. It is the CHFM's responsibility to ensure project completion within budget and on schedule. The healthcare organization depends on the CHFM to safeguard its best interests, including the health of its employees and the productivity and efficiency of the facility. The CHFM is expected to exercise due diligence as a condition of continued employment.

Staffing for Specialized Technical Services

Many technical services are specialized to the point that they require professionally-qualified personnel. University teaching hospitals and other large healthcare organizations may find that they can justify full-time personnel for such positions. Smaller operations may need only a part-time specialist in a particular field. Many companies who have a qualified person on staff assign that person to the task on a part-time basis. If there is no such person on staff, the facility manager may contract with a qualified consultant for intermittent service in each area of need. Such consultants are often paid a "retainer" fee plus an additional amount for actual service. Stipulate in the contract that your facility requires "on-call" emergency service.

Important Terms

- Improvement - An improvement is a change in a facility, system, or equipment that increases the functionality or productivity, enhances the value, or in some way makes the facility, system, or equipment better. An example would be an upgrade to a facility's telephone system.

- Alteration - An alteration is a change in a facility, system, or equipment that enables it to function differently from its original purpose. An example would be changing a group of patient rooms into a treatment area.
- Expansion - An expansion is a change in a facility, system, or equipment that enlarges or expands it. An example would be the addition of a new wing to a hospital.

Maintenance & Operations

Energy Saving

Direct Digital Controls

Direct digital controls make use of microprocessors and sophisticated programming to control a variety of electrical devices. The aim of the digital control is to save energy by not using it at times when specific spaces are closed. Digital controls can turn on and off lights, air handlers, heating units, and ventilation units, according to a preset schedule. Direct digital controls can also be used to enhance temperature management in areas that are not used 24 hours per day. Digital controls can provide a warm-up period in cold weather and a cool-down period in hot weather. Hence, the building or offices are at a comfortable temperature when the staff arrives, without the heating or air-conditioning wasting energy during the unoccupied period.

Alternative Measure

Listed below are alternative measures that can save energy:

- Use direct digital controls that allow different day and night temperature settings
- Draw light-colored drapes over windows during dark hours
- Reduce the usage of incandescent lamps
- Unless needed for treatment areas, limit the use of incandescent bulbs to 200 watts
- Where possible, replace mercury-vapor lights with fluorescent lamps
- Use a time-clock control for outside lights
- Where practical, use motion or infrared sensors to control lights in specific rooms or areas
- When incandescent lamps are necessary, use energy-efficient ones
- Collect rainwater for watering plants
- Reduce glassed-in areas and utilize thermal or double-glazed windows

Quad

Quad means the amount of energy produced, consumed, or held in reserve. It is a very large amount that is equal to one quadrillion BTU. Expressed in terms of oil, a quad is 172.4 million barrels. It also equals the energy produced by 968,900 million cubic feet of natural gas, 38,461,500 tons of coal, or 27,322 pounds of uranium. It would take the entire population of the world working steadily for eight hours a day for 90 days at 100% capacity to produce a quad of energy.

Energy Committee

Effective energy management is not the province of one person or one department, but involves everyone in the organization, from top management to employees at the lowest level. The administrator may appoint Energy Committee members to ensure conservation. The Energy Committee is likely to include a person from each major department or division of the healthcare organization. It may have subcommittees, such as a Transit Committee responsible for shuttles between sites and staff incentives for using public transit. The responsibilities of the Energy Committee are planning and implementing the energy program of the organization. While the energy philosophy should be set by top management, the details of the operation and monitoring of the program are the responsibility of the Committee members.

Energy Management Program Phases

An energy management program should consist of three phases:

- Phase 1 includes energy conservation steps that can be done immediately with minimal inconvenience and disruption. These steps may include adjustments to heating/cooling and lighting, replacements or cleaning of air filters, and improved management of electricity usage.
- After Phase 1 has been implemented and evaluated, the organization can move on to Phase 2, which involves changes in operational practices.
- Phase 3 involves physical changes to the facilities and may require funding from management, and using money saved through the changes of Phases 1 and 2.

Energy Database

An energy database is an important first step toward an energy management program. An energy database helps the CHFM thoroughly understand how much energy is used and how it is used. The database should include records of energy consumption for the organization, broken down by activity and area of the Physical Plant. The CHFM can try to obtain energy records from similar organizations nearby for comparison, or ask the US Department of Energy (DOE) and the EPA for assistance. The DOE's analysis database is at https://apps3.eere.energy.gov/ba/pba/analysis_database/. You organization's database should chart its energy costs, including the percentage of the budget spent on energy. Energy costs can be analyzed according to time period and also by service or activity.

Energy Program Evaluation

The goal of an energy program is to control and reduce energy consumption, thereby reducing costs. The CHFM measures and analyzes the results of the organization's energy monitoring to determine how effective the conservation program is. Measure consumption at the end of each phase of the program or at predetermined intervals. Compare old data with new data over similar time periods, so that data from a warm period when air-conditioning is required is not compared with a cold period when the building must be heated. Use data analysis to establish levels for both variable and fixed consumption. Your Quality Assurance manager can help you with measurements.

Time Clock Energy Control System

Among the four types of control systems for energy management, the time clock is the cheapest and simplest. The system uses a time clock to turn electric equipment and devices on and off at preset times. The timers can be reset manually whenever the need for the equipment or device changes. An example of this usage is the control of outside lighting, although in many businesses photoelectric cells have replaced the time clock for this purpose. The time clock would probably be set to turn the light on at sunset and off at sunrise, and would have to be reset as the times change with the seasons. Consult with your Security manager to find out which high risk areas should always be brightly lit.

Computer Usage in Energy Control

Computer usage in energy control ranges from the very basic computer chip installed in a thermostat to complex systems that control the load cycle on a building air conditioner that maintains different temperatures in separate rooms. Complex systems can be very expensive and may require a mainframe computer. Software for less complex systems that are appropriate for smaller establishments can run on a PC. Speak with your IT manager about combining functions, such as Security, Life Safety, Maintenance scheduling and record keeping on one computer-operated energy system. A combined system may be cheaper to manage, or you may want the redundancy of separate software running on free-standing computers to limit damage by hackers.

Benchmarking in an Energy Plan

The CHFM uses benchmarks to establish a starting point for an energy program or to set goals for the program. Benchmarks can be taken from other facilities of similar size and function or from other departments within an organization. In order to make the best use of benchmarks, the facility manager should be thoroughly familiar with the performance of his facility. One must compare equivalent departments' performance to avoid "apples to oranges" comparisons that are misleading. The CHFM must obtain benchmarks for both the building equipment and the building systems. Biomedical Engineering can supply benchmarks for the medical equipment.

Baseline Energy Audit

Any program intended to reduce the consumption of energy should start with a baseline energy audit. The audit provides a point against which future measurements can be compared in order to determine if consumption is actually reduced and if there is a cost reduction. Facility performance can be compared to similar buildings in comparable climates through the use of Building Owners and Managers Association (BOMA) benchmarking guidelines, available at http://www.boma.org/. When the baseline energy usage is not very different from the benchmark, there is little chance of great improvements. The greater the difference, the more likely a cost savings can be achieved.

Renovation Projects Qualified for Utility Rebate

Many utility companies offer incentive rebates for projects that are energy efficient. Eligible projects often involve the replacement or upgrading of older technology with newer technology that is more efficient. Some examples of projects in which such improvements can be made are:

- Replacing burner control hardware on a boiler
- Installing more efficient heating units
- Installing a more efficient heat exchanger on a chiller
- Replacing older lighting with newer and more efficient lamps
- Installing a more efficient HVAC system

The US Department of Energy also subsidizes renewable energy projects in 10 states. Details are available at http://www.eere.energy.gov/.

Energy Star Program

Energy Star is a joint program of the US Environmental Protection Agency and the US Department of Energy. The Energy Star Web site is at http://www.energystar.gov/, and it states the goal of the Energy Star program is to help Americans "save money and protect the environment through energy efficient products and practices." The Energy Star program encourages energy conservation in private homes and in businesses. Among the strategies for businesses are energy management guidelines, information about sustainable energy design for new buildings, and information about "green" buildings. The strategies offered by Energy Star aid in setting goals, the measurement of current energy usage, and tracking savings from improvements. The program also offers a rating system for energy performance.

Energy Reports

The CHFM measures the energy consumption of a piece of equipment on a periodic basis, so that changes can be monitored and recorded in an energy use log. When the energy use log for that equipment shows a decrease in operating efficiency, it may indicate that something more than routine maintenance is needed. Minor or even major repair may be required in order to return the equipment to its original operating level. In some cases, the decrease in efficiency may be great enough to indicate that it is time to replace the item. If the machine is expensive and still useable, it could be refurbished and moved to an area where it will receive less use and can provide back-up in case the new machine fails.

Maintenance and Repair

Maintenance is the activities necessary for the upkeep of equipment, buildings, and grounds. Maintenance includes inspection, non-janitorial cleaning, painting, parts replacement, and minor repairs. The nature of maintenance is preventive, in that it is intended to prevent breakdowns. Maintenance does not add to the value of an item.

Repair is curative in nature, since it is a response to something that has broken down, worn out, or been damaged. Repair can be either minor or major. Major repairs may prolong the life of equipment or property but should not add to the value of the item.

Maintenance History and Machinery History

Maintenance management should keep two types of records about equipment:

- A maintenance record that is an audit trail showing that maintenance has been done and a record of any problems or failures the equipment has had. The audit trail is a maintenance history that shows that work orders have been issued and that maintenance has been completed. Time required, parts used, and any special problems may be part of the record.
- The machinery history is a record of breakdowns, problems, and repairs, including dates of the problems and repairs. It should also include a description of the problem. Machinery histories are important for the CHFM to use in the decision-making process of whether to repair or replace an item of equipment.

Outsourcing Maintenance Activities

In some situations, it is advantageous for a healthcare organization to hire an experienced maintenance firm, rather than trying to employ an in-house staff large enough and with the variety of skills and knowledge needed for all the Maintenance and Operations tasks. Professional management firms perform the Maintenance and Operations tasks and handle related tasks, such as parts and materials purchases and staffing issues. Professional management firms can also reduce operating costs by securing bulk purchase discounts for items needed by several properties they manage. Professional managers may be more knowledgeable about market trends and impending changes in codes and laws than the in-house staff.

Maintenance and Repair Staffing

Staffing needs vary greatly depending on the size and function of the facilities. For example, a university teaching hospital has hundreds of maintenance workers, whereas a private clinic may contract out its maintenance to a couple of part-time workers. However, some common principles always apply, regardless of the size of the facility:

- Personnel who are technically competent are necessary in all situations
- Staff members should always be full-time unless the size of the operation makes part-time staff sufficient

- Staff should be trained in ways that improve efficiency and technical skills, including how to inspect for deficiencies
- The CHFM should identify leadership qualities in maintenance staff and encourage its development

Even when most of the staff are employed by a professional management firm, some tasks should be performed by in-house personnel. Among them are budgeting, quality control, evaluation, and tasks related to standards and policies.

Grounds Maintenance

The grounds of a facility include paved areas, such as parking, driveways, helipad, and walkways, and landscaped areas of lawn and other plantings. Large facilities usually have both a covered parking deck and an outdoor paved parking lot. Medevac helicopters may land on a ground-level helipad that is in the parking lot or a rooftop heliport. Keep all paved areas and structures clean and clear of debris because the helicopter blades whip it up as projectiles. Make repairs as soon as possible. Efficient planting means choosing perennial plants that resist disease and insects, are drought-tolerant, and do not overgrow and require pruning. Avoid annuals. Mulch to suppress weeds. Choose grass and plants suitable for shade or sun, as the location requires. Install an automatic irrigation system to free staff from watering. Grounds maintenance includes cleaning, mowing and edging, trimming and pruning, fertilizing, and controlling pests.

Maintenance Inventory Control

The Maintenance Department must have various parts and supplies on hand in order to make the repairs and perform the preventive maintenance tasks required of them. Maintenance staff must to be able to quickly ascertain inventory — what is on hand and backordered, how much of a given item, and when a reorder is needed. Maintenance works with Purchasing to control inventory. Many businesses use a software program to track holdings, consumptions, and purchases. An inventory should list each item by name, the number of the part, and how many are in stock. Computerized inventories are only as accurate as the data input and should be confirmed periodically by a physical count of the holdings.

Maintenance Work Order

A work order for the Maintenance Department is a staff member's request for something to be fixed or replaced. Patients and visitors do not complete work orders. The work order notifies the maintenance secretary or dispatcher that something is wrong or has broken and needs attention. The work order identifies the item that needs attention, its location, and the person making the request. It also includes the date and time the request is generated. Some businesses use a printed form with items that can just be checked off when service is needed. Other companies use a form with spaces to be filled in with the problem, location, service requestor, etc. The simplest form of a work order is a verbal request from a department head to the head of maintenance. Verbal requests are usually not tracked and recorded. It is better to have the staff member complete a form so that scheduling and resources can be allocated properly.

Implementation

The Maintenance Department secretary receives the completed work order from a staff member by internal mail, fax, e-mail, or phone-in, and logs it with a time stamp. The secretary alerts the supervisor if there are duplicate requests for the same work, and may phone the requestor to obtain clarification for the Maintenance supervisor and to get the cost center number (if applicable). The supervisor reviews the work order to prioritize it. Work orders are not performed on a first-come-first-served basis. Work orders are prioritized as emergency (something that must be done at once), routine (something that should be done as quickly and efficiently as possible), and backlogged (something that must wait for parts, replacement, or cannot be done right away for some other reason). The supervisor may investigate who can do the work at the lowest cost. The supervisor signs the work order to authorize the work to begin as requested and follows up to ensure it was completed.

Management of Refrigerants

Environmental Protection Agency (EPA) rules require that refrigerants be tracked from purchase to disposal because they deplete the ozone layer of the atmosphere. The CHFM must know Section 608 of the Clean Air Act of 1990, 40 CFR Part 82, Subpart F. Technicians who service appliances that use 50 pounds or more of refrigerant, and the owners of those appliances, must keep invoices showing how much refrigerant was added, along with records of service that indicate date and service type. Maintenance technicians use a computer software package that complies with EPA requirements to track refrigerants (e.g., Enterprise Refrigerant Manager, FX Mobile, and ESS). The facility manager develops a policy for the handling of refrigerants that covers purchases, usage, and reclamation and ensures that the policy is implemented.

Water Heating Systems

The three most common water heater systems are:

- The heater storage tank, which is the least efficient because of inadequate insulation and a low rate of recovery. Heater storage tanks may be used to boost water temperature for washing dishes or in buildings too far from the main heating plant for economical transport of the hot water.
- Heat exchangers, which are very efficient and can provide different water temperatures. Their major disadvantage is that they are used with a steam or hot-water heating system, which reduces their efficiency during the months when heating the building in not necessary.
- Side-arm heaters, which are capable of quickly providing large quantities of hot water. They are moderately efficient. Hot water produced by a side-arm heater can be transferred to a storage tank when production exceeds demand. Careful balancing of the heater output, the capacity of the storage tank, and peak demand for hot water is necessary to maintain efficiency.

Medical Gases

Although an anesthetist or respiratory therapist administers medical gases, Maintenance staff change the cylinders and connect the supply lines. All personnel who handle medical gases must be thoroughly trained to avoid mix-ups that can result in injury or death of a patient. Staff are trained to recognize the various color-coded gas labels they may encounter, the correct method of connecting the cylinders to the delivery system, and the fact that the fittings on the cylinders must never be changed. Storage areas for medical gases should be separate from storage for industrial gases. Whenever a gas container is connected to the delivery system, it should be inspected carefully by a qualified person before the gas from the new container is allowed to enter the system.

Direct and Alternating Current

Direct current (DC) supplies constant volts and amperes when the electric load stays the same. Alternating current (AC) supplies volts and amperes that vary over a time period even when the electric load is unchanged. Some security systems and emergency devices, such as exit lighting, uses direct current, which is usually supplied by one or more batteries. Local utility companies supply alternating current for businesses and for household use. Most of the electricity used in a healthcare facility is of the alternating current type.

Emergency Energy Systems

Healthcare facilities must be able to supply temporary electrical power when there is an interruption in the power from the local utility company. Temporary is defined as 2 hours up to 8 hours. Emergency power generated by the hospital must meet the requirements of the National Electric Code. Power must be available for such functions as minimum lighting and ventilation, Operating Theater, Emergency Room, nurseries, life-support, monitoring equipment, exit lighting in public areas, and technical laboratories. Emergency power for direct current devices may be supplied by a battery system. Alternating current can be produced by an internal-combustion generator that uses either gasoline or diesel oil. An AC generator can supply electricity for several days.

Sprinkler Systems

Wet-Pipe and Dry-Pipe

Both types of sprinkler systems automatically provide water for the suppression of a fire in the protected area. In a wet-pipe system, water is present in the pipes that supply the sprinkler heads at all times. The pipes in a dry-pipe system contain air until a sprinkler head activates, which releases a control valve for the water. Local codes often require the wet-pipe system, but in climates where the pipes may freeze, an antifreeze solution may be necessary during colder weather. In some areas, the codes permit the dry-pipe system in order to avoid the frozen pipe problems.

Sprinkler Head Selection

Sprinkler heads are of different types and can be installed in different ways. When choosing a sprinkler head that is also a heat-sensing device, it is necessary to know the maximum normal temperature of the ceiling on which it will be installed, since the sprinkler head must have a minimum rating that is higher than that ceiling temperature. The CHFM must give attention to the positioning and spacing of the sprinkler heads. Aesthetics may or may not be of concern, depending on the use of the protected space. The sprinkler heads must be appropriate for the area and must be reliable.

Inspection

During the inspection of a sprinkler system, the CHFM or delegate accompanies the Fire Marshal to test the alarms. They check the piping for pitch, leaks, and loose pipe hangers. If an antifreeze solution is used, it is checked for adequacy. Sprinkler heads are checked for anything that could hinder activation, such as dust and mineral deposits. In recently painted areas, the inspectors ensure that paint has not clogged the heads. The system should also be checked for the reliability, capacity, and pressure of the water supply. If the CHFM delegates a staff member to perform sprinkler inspections, then the delegate should have appropriate training and experience and should be knowledgeable about the applicable standards

Fire Suppression Systems

Another water-based system is a misting or fogging system. Foggers are gaining use as a replacement for halon systems, which were phased out by 2000. A fogger system involves a perforated tube installed at the top of the walls of the protected space. One liter of water under high pressure may be adequate to suppress a fire in an enclosed room. Carbon dioxide is a gas that can be used to suppress fires involving electrical equipment, gas, or a flammable liquid. Dry chemical systems use a powder mixture that can extinguish fires in flammable liquids, such as cooking oil. Dry chemicals are preferable for kitchens and heliports.

Fire Detection System

A building fire detection system should not depend on any single element of a fire to cause an alarm, but should be able to detect heat, smoke and radiant energy. Heat detectors may be of the fixed-temperature type, which activates at a preset temperature. Rate-of-rise detectors are activated by the speed at which the temperature rises. Smoke alarms may work through the interruption of the flow of electric energy through ionized air (ionization detectors) or through the disruption of a light beam in a photoelectric detector. Flame detectors are activated by visible radiant energy or flame. Manual alarm stations allow a person who has discovered a fire to activate an alarm.

Water Hardness

Water hardness depends on the amount of calcium and magnesium salts dissolved in the water. Heating hard water causes the salts to precipitate out, which results in a buildup of lime in pipes and on plumbing fixtures. Lime deposits also settle on items washed in the water; for example, hard water spots cloud glassware. The salts mix with some soaps and cleansers to form the sticky substance that sometimes precipitates onto washed items and is known as "soap crud." Hard-water-salt eliminators, such as zeolite, can be used to remove the hard-water salts and "soften" the water. Otherwise, extra cleansers are required to overcome the effects of the salts, which can also damage water heaters, heat-exchangers and boilers.

Upfeed and Downfeed Water Distribution Systems

Both upfeed and downfeed systems are ways to transport water to where it is needed in a building. Upfeed systems are used when the pressure of the water supplied by the water utility is sufficient to supply fixtures throughout a building of up to six floors. A circulating pump may be added to a system when the water pressure from the utility or from a well pump is insufficient to overcome resistance in the piping or the height of the building. Downfeed systems are used in tall buildings. Water is pumped to a storage tank higher than the uppermost fixture in the building, and then flows by gravity to the fixtures on demand.

Water Supply Maintenance Problems

Maintenance workers most commonly deal with dripping faucets and the noise caused by vibration and expansion of the water pipes (water hammer). Dripping faucets waste water and increase needed cleaning which increase expenses. The sound of the dripping water can distract and annoy staff and can be quite disturbing to noise-sensitive patients. The same is true for vibration and expansion noises. Dripping faucets can usually be fixed by changing valve seat washers. Expansion and vibration noise can be reduced by adding pipe insulation, decreasing hot water temperature, and installing expansion devices. Leaking pipes are more serious problem, which may require replacement of pipes or connections.

Biomedical Equipment Technicians

Biomedical equipment technicians (biomedical engineers) are trained to repair, maintain, adjust, and calibrate medical equipment that is electronic, hydraulic, or electromechanical. Their post-secondary education ranges from a technical school degree to a Bachelor of Science in Engineering, along with a significant amount of on-the-job training and specialized medicine courses. However, managers often hold a Master of Biomedical Engineering degree. Their tools include specialized software and computers. The equipment for which are responsible includes imagers (x-ray, ultrasound, and CAT scan machines); voice-controlled operating tables; defibrillators and heart monitors; hospital beds; and electric wheelchairs. Biomedical engineers must be able to work in the presence of patients and to repair an in-use machine without disturbing the patient. Their work hours are irregular and they are expected to share on-call duties.

Roof Maintenance

A hospital roof holds heavy equipment that affects its neighbors, such as a heliport, water tanks, and air conditioning units. Roofs should be inspected regularly and preventive maintenance performed so that small problems can be corrected before they become major ones. The inspector should look for such things as loose mortar and flashing, broken coping, missing flashing, blocked drains, and deteriorated or open joints. Leaves, branches, and other debris should be removed daily if there is a heliport. Small cuts and cracks must be resealed to prevent leaking inside the building. Major repairs are needed if you observe the following: Water ponds; ice damming; delamination of roofing felt; cracked asphalt; or deteriorated coating.

Exterior Walls and Facade Features

The maintenance of the building's exterior is heavily influenced by its geographic location. Urban buildings deteriorate from automobile emissions and industry that create acid rain and smog. Coastal buildings develop a crust of salts and dirt and require extra maintenance. Desert buildings crack from widely fluctuating temperatures and desiccation on a daily basis. Maintenance requirements also depend on the type of material used in the exterior surfaces. Maintenance usually involves cleaning or washing the exterior of the building, and care must be taken to use cleaners and cleaning methods that are appropriate for the materials. The building should be inspected annually for indications of leaking and damage.

Windows and Doors

Windows and interior and exterior doors require regular inspections. Fix problems as soon as possible after they occur to maintain patient safety. Pay particular attention to areas where lab animals are housed and pharmaceuticals are stored. Problems include the disintegration of frames, warping, swelling, and the replacement of weather-stripping. Problems can also arise from the use of inferior materials and poor workmanship. Windows may need the replacement of old putty, trim, or broken sashes, and should be washed at least twice a year in most locations. A quarterly inspection is needed for doors. Dust doors and wash them. Replace damaged frames, glass panes, locks or hardware. Repaint the door in the appropriate color code.

Preventive Maintenance

Preventive maintenance is any activity performed to keep a device or a facility operating properly and to forestall the development of preventable problems. Regular preventive maintenance activities are scheduled at specific intervals and include the inspection of devices, equipment, and facilities. Ad hoc preventative maintenance occurs before a natural disaster, such as boarding windows before a hurricane. Preventative maintenance contributes to cost savings by reducing the need for major repairs and by decreasing work interruptions. Preventive maintenance is vital in a healthcare organization because it ensures that medical equipment is always in proper working order when it is needed.

File the manufacturer's recommendations for a preventative maintenance schedule when you buy a new piece of equipment, and put the suggested date in your tickler file as a reminder. If there is no instruction guide provided when you purchase a second hand machine, ask the vendor to provide one or assign a mechanic or Biomedical Engineer to write a manual as a resource for less skilled workers. Start a maintenance log for each new machine purchased, and keep it for the life of the machine or until its tax depreciation is finished, whichever comes later. Update the log with a description of each maintenance item performed, the name of the maintenance worker, the date and duration of maintenance, along with possible problems and feedback from the maintenance worker. Keep the log readily available with any relevant publications, such as service and operation manuals, and specialized tools for workers' use. Inspection and repair records, inspection schedules, and "as-built" drawings are also among the resources that should be available.

Predictive Maintenance

Predictive maintenance is any activity designed to determine whether or not a piece of equipment is in need of service or repair. The equipment is tested with non-invasive techniques that may include infrared scanning and the analysis of vibrations or of lubricants. When the tests reveal no need for repair or extensive servicing, downtime is avoided, money for service or repair is saved, and the staff can concentrate on items that do need attention. Avoidance of downtime through predictive maintenance is very important to the critical functions of healthcare facilities. Hospitals have a legal Duty of Care and must demonstrate due diligence through predictive maintenance.

Corrective Maintenance

Corrective maintenance is any activity that repairs or restores an item it to its former condition. Corrective maintenance takes place after a problem develops but before the equipment item undergoes a major failure or breakdown. The need for corrective maintenance will arise even when an organization has an excellent preventative maintenance program and all equipment is cared for properly. While much of the minor repair work for a company's various types of equipment may be performed by staff personnel, some items will require the attention of an expert. Items in this category may include elevators, major plumbing or electrical problems, and alarm systems.

Emergency Maintenance

Emergency maintenance is necessary when a situation poses a threat to the life and health of patients and staff. Consider it a type of corrective maintenance that must take place immediately. On-call staff or contractors must respond within the hour. Situations requiring emergency maintenance may result from a fire, severe weather such as a hurricane or flood, criminal activity, or the sudden failure of a major equipment item or system. Examples include an elevator breakdown or a leak in a gas line. Facility managers should plan ahead for emergency maintenance and have in place a plan of action for various types of situations.

Contract Services

Contract services, which are sometimes called vended services, are supplied on a regular basis by outside contractors. The contracts with these vendors include the specifications of the service and the fees. Contracted services may include: Cleaning; security; various types of inspection and routine maintenance; emergency repair and maintenance of essential services; the collection of trash and recyclables; snow removal; plumbing; electrical services; laundry; food vending; the control of rodents and other pests; window washing and other outside maintenance tasks; lawn and grounds maintenance; and heliport management. The healthcare organization awards contracts services after a careful review of the bids from all interested contractors and a reference check for each.

VENDOR SELECTION

The CHFM must evaluate the following criteria before awarding a contract to a service provider who has responded to a Request for Proposals:

- The reputation and references of each bidder — The CHFM may ask if the contractors are bondable and engage an investigations firm to perform a background check. The reference check should include a verbal interview if at all possible, as letters can be falsified.
- Comparison of the services and the proposed prices offered by each bidder —The CHFM determines if the services offered by different contractors are equivalent. The CHFM looks at the size of the firms, the experience they have, the type of clients they have served, their effectiveness, and their methods.

The CHFM awards the contract to the contracting firm that is the best possible fit for the healthcare organization and that offers pricing that does not exceed the healthcare organization's budget.

RFID

Radio frequency identification (RFID) has three major applications in the healthcare industry: Asset management, patient care, and inventory control. An RFID tag contains an integrated circuit that stores information. A Biomedical Engineering technician attaches an RFID tag to equipment so it can be tracked quickly, without staff spending time hunting for it. An RFID can be used as a means of positive identification for a patient, particularly a baby. RFID tags reduce treatment errors and can prevent child abductions. RFID tags are also be used to identify lab specimens to reduce reporting errors. RFID tags are attached to stock items for scanning, so staff can inventory quickly. Hospital staff must maintain adequate stocks, track consumption of drugs, and record installation of surgical devices. The use of RFID tags help to reduce the number of lost and stolen items.

CCTV

Closed circuit television (CCTV) is an important part of a healthcare facility's security system and the tapes are subpoenaed in court. CCTV cameras allow surveillance of common areas, such as parking lots, waiting rooms, exits and other areas where privacy is not an issue. The cameras can deter illegal behavior, since most people are less likely to commit criminal acts when they know they are being watched or recorded. When a criminal act does occur, the cameras can provide legally acceptable evidence and documentation. In some situations, a CCTV system can be used for patient monitoring. Other security uses include monitoring access to restricted areas and employee behavior.

LONG-TERM PREVENTATIVE MAINTENANCE PLANNING

One way of planning for a preventative maintenance program is to construct a maintenance schedule for a full year in advance. The preventative maintenance manager should determine which items of equipment should be serviced weekly, monthly, quarterly, semiannually, and annually. Some equipment may need different maintenance tasks at different time periods, for example, weekly cleaning but daily calibration. All of this information can be built into a work-order schedule, which if followed diligently will ensure that all the preventative maintenance tasks are performed on time. A well designed schedule can help to reduce dependence on overtime and the use of contract workers.

ORGANIZATION FOR MULTI-SITE OPERATIONS

When a healthcare organization has multiple campuses or satellite facilities, the size of the Facilities Department varies with the size and functions of the various locations. It is likely that at least Security, Parking and Custodial Services will be provided for each location. The office of the

Facilities Manager is likely to be at the main campus, and there may be one reception center there that handles work requests for all the locations. Unless the satellite facilities are very large, specialized service personnel and Biomedical Engineers are based at one campus and shuttle to maintain and repair equipment at all the locations. It is quite possible that contracted personnel may be used for much of the work at the satellite locations.

ELEVATORS

CARPET

Materials used for the interior of elevator cars should be easy to clean and not difficult to maintain. A common material used to finish the floor is carpet, because it damps down sounds and absorbs slush in winter. Elevator carpeting should be heavy, with edges that do not curl, roll, or fray easily. The carpet must be removable for cleaning, since it accumulates a great deal of dirt and biohazard soil. Cuts, tears, and frayed edges create a tripping hazard and should be repaired at once. Consider carpet tiles, which are easier and less expensive to replace than an entire carpet.

PROBLEMS WITH GUIDE RAILS AND CABLES

Guide rails are the vertical tracks on which wheels move the elevator car from one floor to another. There is usually no problem with the guide rails, unless the building's foundation has shifted or settled, or construction cracks cause them to get out of alignment. The wheels, however, need lubrication of their bearings and may need to be replaced due to wear. The cables suspend the elevator car. Several redundant cables are attached to the car, although each one is strong enough to support the car. Cables can become worn and frayed and will need to be replaced regularly.

CONTROL SYSTEM

In the 1970s, microprocessor controls started to replace the relays that previously controlled automated elevators. Now, fully computerized control systems are available. A fully computerized system is very expensive to install, but it can be programmed by a manager to minimize waiting time for an elevator, as when the Code Blue team responds to an arrest, or to make the Shabbat elevator stop on every floor on Saturdays. Semi-computerized systems, which make use of standard or limited programs, are also in use. When the CHFM plans a replacement or upgrade of the control system, he or she must consider the age and condition of the current system, the demands placed on the elevators, and the budget. Some updating can be accomplished with an overlay modernization, rather than replacing the entire system.

RELOCATION MANAGEMENT

An example of a small relocation is transferring staff from one office to another. An example of a large move costing more than $1 million is moving an MRI machine. Small relocations are usually handled by the in-house maintenance staff, whereas large moves require the services of a professional moving company. All moves should be planned carefully, so that there is a minimum of disruption to the work of the organization. Ideally, there should be little or no disruption to patient care. The project manager is responsible for scheduling tasks involved in the move. The project manager and millwright make detailed plans well ahead of the move. Supervisors from other trades and Biomedical Engineers may also be involved. Give all personnel written notice of the schedule at least 3 days before the movers begin work.

FOLLOW UP

Whether the relocation is just a change of offices or the relocation of a whole department to a new addition to the facility, there are some follow-up tasks that will be needed. In the first two or three days after a move, maintenance personnel or movers should be available to help with adjustments, such as: Fine-tuning the location of furniture or movable equipment; hanging artwork or patient information posters; and repairing nicks and scratches to furniture. Extra trash pickup may be needed for the removal of packing materials, and the movers should collect the used boxes and cartons. Heavier-than-usual cleaning may be needed for the first few days after the move. Biomedical Engineers, millwrights, and registered technologists adjust and calibrate the heavy medical machinery. IT and the switchboard supervisor must verify that phones and networks are available. Plumbers, HVAC technicians, and electricians verify utilities are working properly.

Employees Involved

The better informed employees are about what to expect, the less traumatic any change is likely to be for them. Inform the employees involved in a relocation about the proceedings before, during, and after the actual move. Plans and schedules should be made carefully, and the information communicated to those concerned. Management should make sure that information about changes in rules and regulations, new addresses and telephone numbers, parking, and food service is shared with all involved employees. Keys and new business cards should be issued. Guidelines for packing up the old location should be issued early enough for all tasks to be completed before moving day. If patients are repatriated or transferred to another unit, work with the Nurse Manager and switchboard supervisor to ensure there is a method of tracking them.

Utility Shutdowns

Utility shutdowns can occur for many reasons. Some are emergency situations, such as a broken water main or a power failure. Healthcare organizations are required to have color-coded emergency plans in place and to rehearse evacuations, decontamination, and fire control. The objectives are to save lives, limit property damage and the spread of disease, and reduce negative impact on patient care. Scheduled shutdowns are not emergencies. They are necessitated by construction, routine maintenance and repairs, testing of generators and fire protection systems, and repairs or adjustments to other building systems. These routine interruptions to utility service are planned and scheduled in advance, so that all affected personnel can be given written notification of what to expect at least 3 days before the interruption.

Repair Costs

Many organizations combine funds for alterations and renovation with funds for maintenance and repair. Unless steps are taken to ensure an adequate percentage of the funds are spent for maintenance and repair, the bulk of the funds may be spent for alteration and renovation projects, since there are usually far more requests for alterations than the available funds can provide. One effective method of control is to set a ceiling on how much can be spent for alterations and renovation. The ceiling can be established as a percentage of the fund or as a dollar amount. Another method is to allocate the funds.

Condition Assessment

A condition assessment is a tool for determining the effectiveness of maintenance and repair and for properly allocating and spending funds. The assessment involves a complete audit of the facility. The work should be done by an outside consultant under the supervision and guidance of the in-house staff. The in-house staff do not usually have the necessary time for such an in-depth analysis and could unconsciously bias the outcome of the study. Consultants for a condition assessment can be provided by many large architectural and engineering firms. Their objective is to lower operating costs and improve the facility condition index (FCI).

Blueprints

Mechanical Views

A set of blueprints will include a separate drawing of each of the mechanical and electrical systems in the building. These drawings are often copies of the plan view with the symbols added that are specific to the indicated system. Systems that will probably require separate views include electricity, plumbing, air-conditioning, heating, closed-circuit television, security, fire protection, and ventilation. Mechanical views are used during the construction and renovation of a building. They can also be used later in analyzing systems for energy efficiency, in planning upgrades to the various systems, and to avoid accidents, such as drilling into wires in a wall.

Use in Maintenance

Detailed blueprints and the written specifications that accompany them contain information that can be helpful to the maintenance staff in several ways. Among the information that can be determined from a review of the blueprints are: Amounts and types of insulation; space for added insulation or the lack thereof; the exact location of wires and pipes within walls, floors, or ceilings; the capacity of the current electrical, heating, water, or ventilation systems; and whether they can support additions. Blueprints can also aid in the planning and scheduling of preventive maintenance. Because of their usefulness, blueprints and specifications should be preserved and filed carefully for the life of the building.

CAD

CAD is computer aided design. Early versions were bulky and very expensive, putting them beyond the reach of most small companies. Today, CAD software exists that can run on a PC and many engineers and architects do their own drawings, rather than resorting to a drafting department. CAD systems can store and recall large amounts of data, aiding in the planning of maintenance and repair. They can also be used to experiment with various ideas about renovation or changes in layout, since the computer can generate pictures of what will happen if a particular change is made. Some CAD systems can produce three-dimensional views and animated walk-through tours of a building. Data stored on a networked system allows access by multiple users.

Sick Building Syndrome

Energy requirements during the 1970s and 1980s resulted in buildings that are airtight, which means that they are designed to allow very little outside air to come into the building. Also, most hospitals keep their windows locked to avoid patient injury or escape. Windows that do not open and air curtains on exterior doors are frequently used to reduce or eliminate outside air. The use of recirculated air inside the building does reduce heating and cooling costs, but also causes a reduction in the quality of the indoor air. The introduction of fresh or outside air is necessary to prevent illnesses among the people working in the building. The Safety Officer and CHFM ensure the proper filters are used to prevent the spread of airborne diseases, such as Legionnaire's and anthrax.

ASHRAE Recommendations for Ventilation

The American Society of Heating, Refrigeration, and Air Conditioning Engineers recommends that outside air be brought into a building at the rate of 900 to 1,200 cubic feet each hour for each occupant to avoid problems with the quality of indoor air,. Properly distributed throughout the building, this amount of fresh air should prevent the problems of sick building syndrome and enable employees to work in a level of comfort that promotes productivity. Patients in a healthcare facility have vulnerable lungs, so Infection Control and Respiratory Therapy may require reverse pressure and other measures in addition to ASHRAE's recommendations, to contain the spread of disease.

Air Filtration

The CHFM must legally provide clean air for employees and patients, according to OSHA and CDC standards. Both outside air and recirculated air should be filtered to remove smoke, grease, chemical pollutants, infectious diseases, aerosolized body fluids, and objectionable odors. Dust and pollens are a problem for allergy sufferers, particularly in Respiratory ICU. Filters are of many types, including HEPA, dry, oil-treated, electronic, and water-spray. The type that is most appropriate for a given situation depends on what substances need to be filtered out of the air. Laboratories have different standards than waiting rooms, for example. Some filters are expensive to install or operate, so the budget is a factor in the filtering decision.

Power Outage

Restarting

Once a power outage is resolved, the healthcare facility needs to get equipment off emergency power and back onto the utility company's electricity as quickly and safely as possible. Maintenance, utility and Biomedical Engineering personnel should be available for the switch-over in case there are problems. Some possible problems arise from a shutdown of more than several hours, and include equipment that has become airbound or has lost calibration or lubricants. Pressure systems may have built up higher pressure because of the lack of demand. As with all interruptions in utility services, take care that there is no loss of essential power for equipment used in patient care. Advise critical areas, such as the O.R. and ICU, to have manual back-ups ready.

Communications

In the event of a utility failure, the CHFM's top priority is informing patient caregivers about what to expect, so patients are not endangered by the sudden failure of life-sustaining or monitoring equipment. Room lighting, blood warmers, hydraulic lifts, imagers and testing equipment are of secondary importance. The avenues of communication the CHFM chooses must be: Reliable; redundant; adequate; timely; and effective. Give caregivers advanced warning of when the interruption is planned, so they can have manual life-support prepared. Let caregivers know when the power will restart, so they can avoid circuit overloads and power surges. The CHFM may use runners and a bullhorn, if absolutely necessary, but avoid alarming patients and visitors.

Scheduling and Installation Coordination

Coordination is basically communication and cooperation between persons working toward a common goal. The facility manager is responsible for working with utility companies, builders, and other contractors to schedule construction and renovation work, and the installation and maintenance of clinical and utility equipment and building systems. The CHFM must work with Emergency Services (the local fire department, police, and ambulance service) Public Health and support agencies in order to ensure the safety of the organization's patients, employees, and property. Coordination communications may be verbal or written. Verbal communications may take place in meetings and conferences and via the telephone. Written communications involves signage, letters, memos, published notices, and e-mail.

Maintenance Manual

The Maintenance Manual contains the departmental Policies and Procedures (P&P). Accreditation surveyors ask to see your up-to-date P&P manual. Human Resources and the Legal Department use it to discipline staff and defend court cases. Review all of the P&Ps in your manual at least once every three years and revise, reauthorize, or archive them as necessary. If your facility does not have a standardized template for P&Ps, use this outline:

- Heading: Date, title, and status (new, revised, or reauthorized P&P)
- Policy: Clearly state the current policy, so Maintenance personnel make consistent decisions in accordance with applicable laws and codes
- Procedure: List necessary equipment, phone numbers, keys, and resource personnel. Number the steps in sequence. Write sufficient detail for seconded Maintenance personnel to perform the work independently, without direct supervision.
- References: List two credible expert resources that are not more than five years old
- Authorization: Sign the policy and obtain the co-signature of a higher authority, if required by law

Operations Manual

The Operations Manual is a formalized statement of your facility's Policies & Procedures. Employee orientation is based on the Operations Manual. Three elements are included in the operations manual: Policies, Procedures, and Forms. Policies are guiding principles for decision making and actions. They tell what is to be done, but do not explain how. Procedures are the step-by-step directions for implementing a policy. They describe an action or procedure in detail. Forms are documents personnel or patients complete, including work orders, purchase orders (PO), request forms, informed consent, and payment authorizations. The manual must be reviewed and updated at least once every three years for accreditation. Keep the information current.

Key Control

Security oversees the key monitoring system to prevent unauthorized key duplication and lending. Keep careful records of keys issued for restricted areas, offices, and controlled access entrances. HIPAA requires that you safeguard confidential patient information. Employees, patients and visitors are entitled to a safe place for their personal belongings. Terrorists can sabotage unlocked utility rooms. Ensure that former employees return their keys at the end of their terms of service. Use a Temporary Key Log to record the name, sign-out date and time, particular area accessed, sign-in date and time, and signature of all people who receive keys. Replace a lock when a key to it is lost. Keys should be stamped with the notation "Do Not Duplicate."

Access Control

Access control systems manage entrance into rooms and areas that are restricted to particular employees. Access control can also be used to lock in an intruder until Security and the police arrive. Access requires a swipe card, proximity card, metal key, entry keypad, or biometric identification. Swipe cards can have magnetic strips, dots, or embedded wire. Proximity cards are used when personnel need to be hands-free, as at a hospital heliport. Key cards can contain a photograph and serve as ID cards. Watermarks or stamps can be included to reduce the likelihood of counterfeiting. Key cards control access to elevators and parking areas, and also control some equipment and lighting. Encourage staff not to leave key cards in their clothing on door hooks because thieves use them to impersonate staff.

Biometrics

Biometrics is a field of biology that deals with the unique features of a person. It includes fingerprints, retinal (eye) patterns, hand prints, voice patterns, and signatures. Biometrics are used in personal identification technology for access control to a facility. Research & Development labs often use biometric systems because they are very secure from competitors, since they provide positive identification of an individual through a "template." The template is a mathematical characterization of a unique feature of an individual. However, the cost of a biometric system currently puts it beyond the reach of most healthcare organizations. The CHFM will probably deal more with swipe cards, metal keys, and keyed entries with access codes.

Problem Resolution with Vendors

When equipment fails because of poor workmanship or faulty parts, it is the responsibility of the facility manager to see that any guarantee or contract terms are fulfilled. Corrective action may include the repair or replacement of the defective equipment. The facility manager may work with the vendor to improve the failure rate of the equipment or part. When it can be determined that the failure rate from a particular vendor is excessive, or if the vendor fails to meet the terms of the contract, that vendor should be dropped by the Purchasing Department.

Important Terms

- Electric demand controller – A system of energy control that permits selected electric devices to operate only within a specified load on the electrical system. The use of the demand controller may cause electricity to be shunted from one device to another device. A device of secondary importance cannot receive power if a top priority device is in operation.
- Demand meter – A special meter that records peak energy requirements for a building. The meter can register kilovolt-amperes or kilowatt demand for a specific time period. The most commonly used time period is a quarter-hour. Once the meter is read, it can be reset to record another energy peak.
- Watt – A measure of electrical energy usage that equals the power developed in a circuit when a current of one ampere flows through a potential difference of one volt.
- Kilowatt – 1,000 watts.
- Kilowatt hour – The use of one kilowatt for one hour.
- Ampere – The standard unit used to measure the rate at which an electric current flows through a device, used to rate electric motors and many electronic devices. Even very small numbers of amperes are dangerous to living bodies.
- Volt – Electrical potential unit, the pressure that allows the flow of electric current.
- Trap – A U-bend in the drain pipe from a plumbing fixture, which holds water and prevents sewer gases from flowing through the fixture into the building.
- Soil Pipe – A waste drainpipe, which can handle all the drainage from a building, including human waste from the toilets.
- Storm drain – A drain for the specific purpose of collecting the runoff from roofs and parking areas. Often, the storm drain does not combine with sanitary drains and cannot lead into a private system for sewage disposal.
- Sewage ejector – A system for pumping waste from plumbing fixtures located below the level of the sewer line for a building.
- Blueprint – A drawing or series of drawings that show the layout of a building, room, plot of land, or the construction of an object. Building blueprints use specific symbols to indicate features such as doors, windows, and electrical outlets.
- CADD – Computer-aided design and drafting uses special software that can save time and money in the production of engineering drawings. AutoCAD is a commonly used program.
- Plan view – A blueprint drawing that shows the space or object as if the viewer were looking down at it from above.
- Elevation view – A drawing showing an outside wall of a building.

Finance

Body-Shop Contracting

"Body-shop" contracting is a type of outsourcing in which the contractor supplies personnel who possess the needed skills and abilities, along with front-line supervision, and the facility manager provides organization, direction, and evaluation. In this situation, the facility manager sets policy, develops requirements, and provides oversight of the work performed by the contracted personnel. Consultants may be able to suggest policy and requirements, but suggestions are subject to the approval of the in-house management. The "body-shop" arrangement provides flexibility through the use of a mix of contracted personnel and in-house staff.

Management Contract

A management contract is used when an organization outsources the management of its facility. The contract creates an agency relationship between the organization and the Maintenance and Operations contractor. The specific rights and responsibilities of both parties should be stated clearly in the contract, so it must be vetted by legal counsel. The contract should detail the duties of the contractor and specify the methods and frequencies of the work. The contract should contain a confidentiality agreement and a statement that all the work is to be in compliance with the laws at the local, state, and federal levels.

Indefinite Quantity Contract

An indefinite quantity contract allows the facility manager to order services or supplies within a fixed dollar amount, but does not limit the deal to a specific contractor. An indefinite quantity contract is most often used for repair work to walls, ceilings, flooring, carpet, glass and concrete for which the maximum square feet is specified. Appliance repair and replacement, painting, and the pruning and removal of trees are other possibilities. When the CHFM determines the need for one of the services or supplies listed above, he or she writes a delivery order against the contract and Accounting obligates the funds.

Job Order Contract

The major use for a job-order contract is for work that exceeds a price that has been specified beforehand. The job-order contract features a price book, which lists prices for specific tasks that have been previously established and agreed upon. When work is to be done under the contract, the number of work units and the price are established by the contractor and the facility manager or contracts coordinator. Then Purchasing places an order for the work. Job-order contracts are advantageous to the medical facility because they allow for a quick response to a need.

Payback Period

Calculation

The payback period is a method of calculating how long it will take a project to pay back the capital investment required for it. The calculation may be used to determine if a project is acceptable or to decide which project is the most acceptable. The payback period is calculated by dividing the cost of the project by the annual net cash flow the project is expected to bring in. If the number of years determined by the calculation is equal to or less than a predetermined figure, the project is acceptable. When calculations are made for the purpose of choosing between two or more projects, the choice would be the one with the shortest payback period.

Advantages and Disadvantages

Among the advantages of the payback period evaluation method is that it is simple to calculate, easy to understand, and simple to use. These factors make it the most popular method of evaluating a capital investment. Both the average payback period method and the actual payback period method provide a measure of risk. However, there are drawbacks to both methods. Both are simplistic and do not give full consideration to the timing of the cash inflow during the payback period, nor do they consider the continued inflow of cash after the payback period. Because of these drawbacks, other evaluation techniques should also be used in the decision-making process.

Average and Actual Payback Periods

The average and actual payback period calculations help the CHFM to make a decision about the acceptability of a proposed project. The average payback period is calculated by dividing the net investment of the project by the expected average annual cash inflow. The actual payback period is a similar calculation that divides the initial investment by the net cash income. The net cash income is the after-tax amount of the savings from the project, plus the depreciation expense tax write-off. The actual payback period considers the timing of cash flows, whereas the average payback period does not.

Life-Cycle Costing

Life cycle costing is a method of determining the acceptability of a project or of deciding between projects by calculating the cost of the project throughout its life. The calculation must include the initial investment, the costs of operation and maintenance, administrative expenses, finance charges, the consumption of energy, and expected modifications and replacements. The CHFM must also consider the final retirement or disposal of the project. In terms of a building, life cycle costing can be expressed as the funds required to build it, operate it, and dispose of it.

Budgets

Operating Budget

The operating budget for a facility is a summary of all projected income and expenses for a specific time period. Operating budgets are often constructed on a monthly basis and include projections for the year. Seasonal expenses, such as lawn mowing and snow removal, must be included. Fluctuations in such items as payroll, administrative expenses, prices for materiel and supplies, taxes, insurance, and general costs must be forecast as accurately as possible. The budget should be reviewed monthly by the facility manager and Accounting, and at least quarterly by a member of upper management. Discrepancies between the budgeted amount of a line item and the actual cost should be investigated and revisions made as necessary.

Formulation: Senior management and departmental managers negotiate and prepare the operating budget. The operating budget team considers both corporate guidelines and forecasts of departmental activity. Each department forecasts the demand for its services, but the priorities that must be met are primary care, hospitalizations, surgeries, births, and emergency care. Forecasts are drawn from market trends, past history, and executive judgment. The team evaluates trends in resource prices and the cost of in-house personnel versus contractors. Purchasing and Human Resources provide the statistics for these forecasts.

Maintenance and Repair Budget

The maintenance and repair budget is part of the operating budget. It covers both routine and preventive maintenance and the custodial care of the facility. The budget must provide cost estimates for both materials and labor needed for the care of the: Grounds; both the exterior and interior of the building; elevators; systems, such as electrical, HVAC, and telecommunications; office technology; Security; Life Safety; furniture; signage; and food service areas. Custodial functions, such as janitorial services, trash removal, pest control, carpet and window cleaning are also part of the maintenance and repair budget.

CONSTRUCTION

Major construction projects are part of the capital budget. Since many capital projects are multi-year projects, the estimated figures for materials, labor, and other line items may change as details of the project are worked out. It is difficult for the CHFM to project costs for employee downtime and supervision until completion of the project without constant input from the project foreman and the Project Manager. The budget must include projected costs for construction, purchase of furnishings, installation, and the warehousing of materials and tools. The most accurate way for the CHFM to prepare the budget is to break out work items and sub-items and list the projected cost for each one.

CAPITAL BUDGET

The capital budget is not discrete for a single year, since construction and renovation may be multi-year projects. Tax laws and company policy control which items can be capitalized. Company policy may establish that single purchases costing less than a predetermined amount may not be capitalized. Line items in the capital budget are projects that are individually justified, and their supporting documentation is part of the budget. Some capital projects may reduce costs of one type while increasing others, such as the replacement of a leased building with one owned by the company. Reflect the findings of your needs analysis for construction and replacement, which is part of your strategic planning, in the capital budget.

UTILITIES BUDGET

The utilities budget is part of the operational budget and contains estimated costs for electricity, water, and heating fuels (oil and gas). Planned energy savings may also be indicated. The facility manager must justify directed purchases, since utilities are often secured from a local, sole-source supplier. Base estimated costs for the various utilities on your facility's historical usage. Utility companies can usually help with these figures, since many have software that can produce sophisticated analyses and accurate forecasts that take into consideration factors such as rate increases and abnormal weather patterns.

FORMULATION

The budget for the facility management department is often the second largest for the organization. It also has unique characteristics that require the CHFM to give explanations and justifications to the Finance Department. The diversity of the facility management budget creates questions because it encompasses widely different areas: Space planning; Waste Management; Security; Housekeeping; mail distribution; and utilities. Government regulations strongly impact the facility management budget, since it is often difficult to determine the cost of compliance. Allow leeway in the facility management budget for reaction to natural disasters and emergencies.

CHARGEBACKS

Chargebacks are a cost control system in which the cost of facility services requested by a department is charged to that department. Chargebacks may be limited to work that exceeds a set standard. One advantage of the chargeback system is that it encourages awareness of costs, and so may lead to lowered operating costs. Department managers may object that:

- The facility manager sets arbitrary rates
- Costs are difficult to calculate and justify
- Chargebacks create conflict with line managers

The facility manager may complain that a chargeback system means a lack of any discretionary budget. It is best for the organization to fund basic needs, and charge departments back for extraordinary usage.

Energy Consumption Records

Instruct your Chief Engineer to verify the energy consumption records for your healthcare facility before you authorize Accounts Payable to pay the utility bills. Energy consumption meters are read at least once a month, and depending on the utility and the organization, they may be read as often as daily. Some utility companies use minicomputer electric meters; others use radio transmission meters. Some companies will provide daily readouts or may grant the facility direct access to the minicomputer readout. Regardless of how your utility company obtains its billing information, keep your own careful logs of your facility's consumption for comparison. Compare current records with logs from previous years or with benchmarks to reveal whether or not energy conservation efforts are successful.

Energy Reduction Goals

The Energy Committee can use your energy consumption logs to develop energy reduction goals for the whole facility. Energy reduction goals must be both realistic and practical for each department in your facility. Departments that have low energy requirements may be unable to reduce their consumption much further. Remind the Energy Committee members to base their goals on reducing energy consumption by a percentage of current usage, rather than on the total cost of energy. Do not allow zealous consumption reduction to interfere with patient care and the quality of test results. Remember that the medical field is competitive, and staff retention is best for patient care and the training budget. If your staff is made uncomfortable by excessive demands for cost reductions, they make seek employment elsewhere.

Load Cycling Systems

A load cycling system is a type of energy management control. The load cycling system staggers operation of large energy-using devices so they do not all operate concurrently. The load cycling system can also be programmed to allow only selected devices to operate during specific time periods. Limiting when and for how long a particular device is in operation controls its energy consumption. One example of load cycling is operating a room's air conditioning unit only when the room is in use. While the air conditioner is operating, shut off another device which is not vital at that time.

Electric Demand Controllers

An electric demand controller is an energy consumption control that is similar to a load cycling system, in that it works with a preset energy requirement. The electric demand controller allows several electro-mechanical devices to operate concurrently until the energy use reaches a preset level. When the preset point is reached, one of the operating devices must be shut off before any additional device can start operating. Electric demand programs are an available part of most computer control systems. Electric demand programs can be very complex and require a large amount of input from management.

Service Contract Elements

The service contract should be written, not verbal. The service contract must identify all parties to the agreement. Clearly state the service to be performed. Specify where the service is to be performed and the frequency of performance. List the service standards to be met. Specify exactly how performance will be measured and the consequences of non-performance or poor performance. Include the date when the contract takes effect its expiration. State whether you will accept subcontractors. Identify costs according to time period, such as hourly or weekly. Cover any special provisions, including security, confidentiality, insurance, how emergencies will be handled, and if overtime will be permitted. Outline circumstances under which the contract can be terminated. All parties to the contract must sign it. Ask your facility's legal counsel to vet the language of your draft before presenting the contract to your service provider.

Evaluation Criteria for Bids

Involve you facility's staff and the Procurement Office in the bid process. The criteria used to select a bid for goods or services are:

- The lowest responsive bid, which may be used for reorders, name-brand items, and other routine situations
- The lowest evaluated bid can be selected from a group of vendors who have been rated and meet a minimum technical score.
- Before a selection is made according to the highest evaluated bid, the vendors are rated and those scoring below a preset level are eliminated. Those remaining are reevaluated, and the contract is awarded to the contractor judged best all-around.

Bidder Qualification Questionnaire

Include the following questions in a bidder qualification questionnaire:

- What year was your company established or incorporated?
- Is your company public or private?
- Has your company ever filed for bankruptcy?
- How many employees work for your company and what are their categories?
- Do your employees have a collective bargaining unit?
- Has your company has ever had a contract terminated?

Do not leave your facility vulnerable to risk. Insist that the bidder supply the following information to qualify for consideration:

- Resumes for key personnel proposed for the project
- Information on completed projects similar to the one now proposed
- Current contracts for building supplies
- Customer references
- Financial references
- Proof of bonding and insurance coverage

Administration

Policies

Policies are the principles of your facility. They must comply with medical ethics, government laws, and professional regulations. Policies are found in the facility's Operations Manual and in each departmental manual. A departmental policy must not conflict with an operational policy. If a conflict is found, then the operational policy takes precedence. Informal verbal policies are passed as stories from one employee to another. Formal, written policies are preferred because they are easier to disseminate and understand. Accreditation surveyors will ask to see your P&P manuals to renew your facility's license. The facility manager sets policies for Maintenance. Policies usually deal with personnel concerns, such as hours of work, benefits, overtime, vacation, sick leave, and grievances. They are also incorporate company rules and quality standards.

CMMS

A CMMS is a computerized maintenance management system. The CMMS contains detailed, descriptive and visual instructions for maintenance tasks. CAD 3D drawings, graphic images, schematics, cut-away diagrams, photographs, illustrations, 2D diagrams, and parts lists from manuals are scanned into the CMMS, provided such copying does not infringe copyright. The drawings support specific directions for exactly how a maintenance or repair task is to be performed. CMMS information is invaluable for less experienced workers. When any worker is seconded during an emergency or labor shortage, the CMMS helps him or her to deal with an unfamiliar item. The CMMS can collect and preserve maintenance and repair information for new and outdated equipment.

Fund Allocation for Projects

Capital projects are given a priority ranking after a careful in-house review. Capital projects are chosen on the basis of:

- Long-range plans
- Expected improvements in the costs of operation
- Changing needs
- Changes in Policies & Procedures
- New technology
- Equipment that needs to be replaced or updated
- Changes in rules, regulations, or standards from governmental or standards organizations
- Changes in business conditions

The Board of Directors deals with major issues arising from the in-house review and makes any final choices before approving the capital budget.

Capital Equipment Purchases

The purchase of capital equipment should be justified and should fit into the organization's total program. Individual items may be grouped with others that are related to the same objective and together they are approved as one project. Among the factors that can justify equipment purchases are maintaining the condition of the facility and replacing or updating equipment in a manner that is cost-effective. New equipment may be mandated by: A new program; a revision of regulations or standards; energy conservation efforts; environmental concerns; efforts to improve efficiency; and desired improvements in costs and labor.

Long-Range Improvement Plan

A long-range improvement plan is also called a long-range capital investment strategy. It is a guide to facility construction and renovation over a period of five to 10 years. The long-range improvement plan helps senior management to understand the issues and priorities facing the organization. It helps accountants and legal counsel keep the facility's investments in line with the strategic plan of the organization. It can also be used to inform the employees and other stakeholders about the organization's long-range goals and priorities. The long-range plan should be dynamic and allow for changes and adjustments because needs and conditions change and individual projects must be eliminated or revamped.

E-Health

E-health means using the Internet and related technologies to improve the collection, storage, and dissemination of medical information. Your organization's Web site is often the initial point of contact for patients and prospective employees and contractors. It is critically important that the Maintenance portion of the Web site be kept up-to-date with announcements of downtime and restarts, construction, and requests for tenders. Employees and physicians need constant access to their computers for continuing education, online diagnostic programs, referrals, and consultations. Laptops with wireless modems are increasingly used for recording patient information, but present a security problem because they are easily stolen and confidential data can be hacked.

Impact of Reconfiguration on Equipment Needs

As hospitals and other healthcare organizations update and modernize their facilities, there is often some effort to consolidate and realign clinical services. Some departments may be downsized, and many procedures and treatments may be shifted from a specialized area to the point of care. Procedures that once required several days of hospitalization can now be done on an outpatient basis, which has reduced the need for beds and associated equipment. An example of this is childbirth: In the 1980s, mothers and babies were retained for five days, but since the mid-1990s they are only retained for a few hours after birth. Diagnostic equipment is more in demand and the equipment has become smaller and mobile, which has encouraged the shift in the location of procedures.

Equipment Evaluation to Predictive Maintenance

Predictive maintenance (PdM) means monitoring the condition of equipment to identify faults before they develop into major problems. PdM is also called condition-based maintenance. Early identification of developing problems enables the Maintenance staff to order parts as needed, rather than carrying unnecessary inventory. Repairs can be scheduled so as to minimize disruptions in service, and sudden breakdowns can be avoided. Maintenance is timed before the machine loses performance and for when it is most cost-effective. Among the tools available for predictive maintenance, perhaps the most important are the eyes and ears of the Operations staff. Their familiarity with a machine or system allows them to notice subtle changes in its condition.

Value Engineering

Value engineering was invented by Lawrence Miles of General Electric Company in 1940 to increase production of B24 bombers for the war effort when not enough traditional materials could be found to complete them as designed. It is now a widely-accepted management tool for lowering cost by substituting equivalent materials that will do the same job without degrading the quality, lifespan, features, appearance or use of a machine. The same requirements for quality, performance, reliability, and safety must be met. Value engineering is a systems-oriented approach with a life-cycle orientation that relates value received to the functions and resources designated for a project.

The value engineering assessment is performed by a team with experience in design, construction, and facility management. Value engineering is also called value analysis or value control.

EPS

Engineered Performance Standards (EPS) were invented at the Department of Defense in the 1950s to deal with maintenance of ageing, war-damaged buildings. EPS requires the CHFM to calculate the allowed number of hours in which a qualified worker, who has average skills and makes an average effort, can produce a predetermined quantity of work. The standards also require good supervision. In order for the standards to be accurate, the facility manager must have an exact knowledge of what is to be done and of any specifications that must be met. Information may come from the facility manager's observations and previous experience, from the manufacturer of equipment that is to be installed or maintained, or from an experienced tradesperson.

Engineered Performance Standards

The CHFM must have a precise and definitive description of the work to be done before trying to calculate engineered performance standards (EPS). The CHFM writes out in detail the exact repair or maintenance task, rather than using a catch-all phrase, such as "fix leaky faucet." Follow this guideline for every EPS you calculate:

- Identify the work location and state how to gain easy access
- Specify the number and type of personnel required for to complete the task
- Indicate the time required to retrieve supplies and for any travel
- Write the standards at an appropriate level for a professional tradesperson who is skilled, possesses the necessary tools, has access to the needed supplies and equipment, and who can be present at the work location when the work is to be done

Scheduling

The facility manager is responsible for allocating personnel, equipment, and materials for specific jobs at specific times. The CHFM schedules work successfully over a three-month block by anticipating what needs to be done and when. The CHFM is flexible and allows a space cushion for delays caused by weather, absent workers, unanticipated changes, and emergencies. Long-term scheduling is required for all large projects, which may span years. Short-term scheduling is for projects that require at least 24 work hours to complete. Weekly scheduling is a plan for the coming week, and includes only jobs for which the availability of materials has been confirmed.

Purchasing Responsibilities

The facility manager is responsible for controlling all departmental Purchase Orders (PO). A Purchase Order is a legally binding contract between the hospital and the supplier, which authorizes the supplier to ship goods and guarantees that the hospital will pay the agreed-upon price. The CHFM must review and approve each PO before the order is placed with the supplier. The CHFM must show due diligence to the Purchasing and Finance departments, by ensuring items are purchased at the best prices and that unnecessary purchases are not made. The CHFM can only authorize purchases from approved suppliers. If an approved source does not already exist, the CHFM locates an appropriate supplier and gets it authorized by the Purchasing manager. Authorized Purchase Orders should be used for all purchases, except when an emergency creates a threat to life or property.

Allocated Funds, Committed Funds, and Expended Funds

Allocated funds are money set aside for a specific purpose. Allocations may be made periodically, such as quarterly, so that the entire budget cannot be spent in the first few months of the year.

Funds are committed when an order is placed. Once committed, the money cannot be shifted to another purpose without negotiation, arbitration, or legal action. When the check is written to pay for the order, the funds are expended. The facility manager must know which of these three types of funds are reflected in a budget report. The facility manager tracks expenses on a spreadsheet, such as Lotus or Excel, or the software program designated by Accounting.

BUDGET REVIEWS AND REPORTS

The CHFM controls the Maintenance Department budget by periodic reviews with an accountant and a senior administrator. The budget for capital projects should be formally reviewed each month. The annual Maintenance budget should be informally reviewed at 6 and 9 months, so there are no surprises at year-end. Additional reviews are needed during the last quarter of the budget year if funds are reprogrammed. Monthly budget reports should provide quick and easily understood information to the facility manager. Monthly reports should reflect the priorities of the Maintenance Department. Pie charts and bar charts allow the CHFM to quickly see whether or not the actual expenditures reflect the departmental plans and intentions.

PROJECT PRESENTATIONS

The CHFM makes presentations for proposed projects to decision-makers, such as the CEO and CFO. The CHFM must remember that the decision-makers are not engineers and must not use jargon. Explain all technical terms. Concentrate the presentation on one major construction project or some type of improvement to the facility or its operation. However, you must also present an alternative to your proposed project. Prepare a formal presentation designed to sell the project. Rehearse thoroughly before presenting your proposal. Use audio-visuals and hand-outs. Be prepared to answer questions, clarify facts and estimates, and explain any point that is not clearly understood by the decision-makers. Be able to cite at least two credible references for your proposed change. If possible, offer to take the decision-makers to a similar facility that has already made the same change, so they can see it completed.

AIDS TO MAKING PRESENTATIONS

Project presentations are greatly enhanced by the correct use of visual aids. However, do not keep the room darkened for more than 20 minutes, as your audience may doze. If you do not have access to an overhead projector, use a flip chart with printed handouts and reproductions of a CAD drawing. Avoid 35 mm slides, if possible. Use slide shows to illustrate a presentation or to give the audience a look at projects or facilities that are similar to your proposal. When the project involves a new concept or new technology, build a 3D mockup. Even though a mockup is expensive, it is quite helpful in explaining a complicated or unfamiliar matter. Mockups can sometimes be supplied by a vendor.

TRAINING

Even licensed employees need training in the details of the work they are expected to do and in the general Policies & Procedures of your organization. Teach both the purpose and procedures when you perform job training. When you update a procedure, hold an in-service training session. Before you put a new piece of equipment into service, schedule operations and maintenance training on it for all employees who will be involved with it. Inform new hires about the type of behavior your hospital expects. Discuss absences, accidents, benefits, and sexual harassment. In the healthcare field, many employees who do not work directly with patients or clients must sometimes deal with them. Give your Maintenance employees sensitivity training for these situations. Explain to your employees that training not only enables them to perform better in their current jobs but can enable them to qualify for promotions.

Large medical organizations have a Training & Development office, which is usually part of Human Resources. Orientation and sensitivity training is entrusted to Training and Development. However, training that is specific to a job or department should be done by the supervisor or manager of that department because he/she is a subject matter expert (SME). The trainer needs to be thoroughly familiar with the job and must be able to observe and evaluate the performance of the employees. The CHFM must compare what an employee is currently doing with what he should be doing (the Engineered Performance Standards). The CHFM should also be able to determine why an employee is performing below his capability. In the facility management area, the facility manager is responsible for technical training and performance appraisals. If you need help providing feedback to an underperforming employee, ask your HR rep to accompany you at the meeting.

Warranties and Guarantees

The facility manager is responsible for ensuring the terms of a warranty or guarantee are fulfilled. The CHFM deals with vendors and ensures that delivery dates and other specifications of purchase contracts are met. Careful record keeping lowers the risk of a warranty being voided on the basis of poor maintenance. File all warranty records. Either use your facility's CMMS, or keep a tickler file to prompt you to schedule equipment maintenance on time. The tickler file helps reduce the costs associated with a piece of equipment by ensuring it is serviced according to the terms of its warranty. Include the expiration date of the warranty on the CMMS or tickler card.

Interdepartmental Cooperation

The Facility Department offers support and maintenance services to the entire healthcare organization, so it is vital for the CHFM to communicate and cooperate with all departments. For example, the CHFM must have access to the OR schedule in order to schedule Housekeeping staff to clean the Operating Rooms appropriately. Other departments must keep the Facility Department informed about their needs for patient-related services, changes needed for heating and air conditioning, and problems with medical equipment. On the other hand, the rest of the establishment must be informed when major repairs or maintenance activities are scheduled.

Work Control Center

The work control center is the central clearinghouse where all maintenance and repair work is coordinated, prioritized, planned, and scheduled. The work control center also handles cost estimates for work requests. The work control center provides a telephone number to staff, where an operator receives requests for service from the entire establishment. The job of the work control center operator is to: Handle complaints, track backlogs, manage emergencies, control the parts inventory, and dispatch materiel and supplies. The CHFM coordinates work for extraordinary situations, oversees inspections for quality control, and evaluates work performance.

Maintenance Deficiencies

When you identify a maintenance deficiency, generate a work order for corrective action. Prioritize the work order according to the severity of the problem. Cross-reference it as a Quality Control correction in a computerized suspense file, which is automatically updated when the task is completed. Identify the cause (or causes) of the deficiency for the Quality Assurance manager. Outline your corrective action so the cause will not engender a cycle of deficiencies and corrective measures. Track trends in deficiencies, so that long-term corrective measures can be put in place. Notify other applicable managers, if necessary.

Engineering Assessment

A detailed engineering assessment is used to identify noncompliance with codes and other Physical Plant problems that can have a negative effect on the organization. An engineering assessment includes electrical, plumbing, HVAC, fire safety, structural and all other building systems. The engineering assessment should also take into consideration the age of the building, its functional layout, and wayfinding measures. Include any future plans for alterations or reconfigurations in the present assessment, since it is not uncommon for a physical structure to become obsolete for its current function, while still being physically usable.

Mechanical System Hygiene

Many modern buildings have sealed windows to prevent heat loss. In medical facilities, windows are also sealed to protect patient confidentiality and to prevent patient abduction or escape. Therefore, the only sources of air are the mechanical and HVAC systems. Keep these systems clean to prevent sick building system and the spread of airborne diseases. Dirty filters become a source of indoor air pollution. Dust, dirt, rust, and other matter can accumulate in the air passageways. Water droplets from humidification or from condensation can stagnate if air is not constantly circulated. The combination of stagnant water, darkness and grime provides an ideal environment for the growth of mold and bacteria. Air passing over these growths becomes contaminated and can cause serious problems in patients, clients, and employees who are allergic and, when the contamination is severe enough, even to those who are not allergic.

Responsibilities During Construction Projects

During a construction project, the facility manager is responsible for seeing that the work is completed properly. The CHFM ensures that plans are followed, that legal requirements are met, that the work is done on time, and that the project stays within budget. At the beginning of the project, the CHFM is responsible for receiving the certificate of insurance and any bonds from the general contractor, and for ensuring that all required permits are on-site. During the construction phase, the facility manager reports at least every other week to senior management concerning the project's progress, any problems, and costs, including those for change orders. The CHFM must secure from senior management any needed approvals. The CHFM is also responsible for seeing that bills are paid by Accounts Payable or Payroll when they are due.

Green Buildings

Green or sustainable buildings are designed, constructed and operated in an ecology-friendly and resource-efficient manner. The design of a green building is intended to: Protect the health of users; increase their comfort; improve worker productivity; use natural resources more efficiently than a conventional building; and reduce the overall environmental impact of the building. Green building practices include: Making use of existing plants and features of the site; using recycled materials wherever possible; optimizing the use of natural light; and using alternative and renewable sources of energy. A thermally-efficient shell, coupled with high-efficiency lighting and HVAC systems, contribute to the green rating of a building. Green buildings use sustainable building materials where possible.

Recycling

Recycling is important, both as an ecological consideration and a possible source of income. Concern for natural resources, conservation, and other environmental issues has become more widespread, so recycling is likely to grow in importance. Among the products a healthcare facility might recycle are: Paper (excluding unshredded confidential documents); glass that is not contaminated with potentially infectious organisms; aluminum cans and other metal; and

Styrofoam and other plastics. A recycling program is likely to require at least a half-time waste manager to set up the program and get it underway. Another initial cost is containers (blue boxes and hoppers) for the recycled materials. Storage and personnel to sort the materials will be ongoing costs.

Wellness Room

The wellness room is a recent concept in patient rooms. It is a modular design that incorporates proven therapies with patient satisfaction to create a flexible, efficient, and comfortable room that is task-centered and of high quality. Wellness LLC makes a turnkey wellness room total package that can be installed quickly in both new constructions and in renovations. The unit includes a bathroom, walls that have electrical wiring already installed, lighting, vinyl finishes, an in-room nurse's station, and furnishings. The comfort of the patient's family has been taken into consideration in the design of the wellness room.

Personnel Recruitment

The CHFM must comply with equal opportunity and affirmative action laws when advertising, screening, interviewing, and selecting new staff for the Facility Department. If you are unsure about how to proceed, contact Human Resources for help. Write the job description in sufficient detail, so that the duties, responsibilities, and requirements can be understood clearly by all applicants. List the requirements for education, licensure, and experience explicitly. Screening means a review of the applications and verification of the data. Your Human Resources officer can arrange a background check of the short-listed applicants for criminal activity and for credit and driving records. Drug testing may also be part of the screening process, since the person you hire will work near pharmacy cupboards around a vulnerable population.

Departmental Strategic Planning

Strategic plans are the long-range plans that set the direction in which the company will move in the next several years. The plans for the Facility Department should fit well with the overall plans for the company. Strategic plans affect decisions concerning renovations versus new construction, the focus of investments, and customer services. Information for strategic planning comes from many sources, including the general policies and the business plan for the corporation, the planning done by the business units, and the history of the corporation. Issues that should be addressed by the strategic plan include: Capacity: relocation and expansion: life-cycle costing: and the capital budget.

Information Sources About Service Contractors

One important source of information about service contractors is other facility managers in your area. Talk to other facility managers you meet at conferences and professional organization meetings. They will be able to supply the names of contractors and comment on their dependability, and the quality and pricing of the contractors' work. Equipment manufacturers sometimes supply maintenance or repair for their own products at their service shops. Their services may be available on a contract basis or through an "as needed" plan. Some engineering and construction businesses provide services, including emergency repairs. Directories and printed and online telephone listings are other sources for the names and addresses of contractors to whom a facility manager might want to submit a Request for Proposal.

Exchange Partners

The group of stakeholders and exchange partners is much more complex for a healthcare organization than for many other businesses. Of all the exchange partners, patients should be considered the most important. Their families and friends accompany them and often serve as informal caregivers. Insurers and fiscal intermediaries are essential, since they provide the highest percentage of a HCO's revenue. Insurers include government programs, such as Medicare and Medicaid, and employers. Regulatory and licensing agencies must be counted as exchange partners, as must quality improvement organizations. These local agencies are your exchange partners: EMS (fire, police, and ambulance); Public Health; utilities; and charity organizations.

Prioritizing Programs

The CHFM can create a matrix that allows different programs to be compared and rated on the same factors or criteria. The CHFM can then prioritize the programs because they are "on a level playing field". The matrix can present a graphic summary of the facility planning issues involved, separated from the space and other deficiencies that should be factored into your decision. Planning issues include: Workload: layout: problems with locations: scheduling: issues with equipment and technology: appearance: problems with building systems: and code problems. Space issues include: Patient rooms: treatment and diagnostic areas: staff and support space: registration and waiting areas: and food service.

Safety Plan

A written safety plan is an effort to reduce accidents and create a safer work environment. In order for the plan to accomplish its purpose, it must be supported by management, and the employees must be convinced of its worth. The safety plan should be part of employee training. Enforce safety policies and procedures consistently. Reward safe working behavior with positive reinforcement (awards, public praise, bonuses, and promotion). Report accidents on a standardized form approved by Employee Health, such as the Department of Industrial Accidents form. Review the form with the Safety Officer before taking action to prevent more accidents of a similar nature.

Safety Committee

Management involves employees in the safety plan and programs by forming a Safety Committee, whose members assume responsibility for:

- Establishing guidelines for safe conditions and behavior
- Collecting employee input for use in establishing training programs for safety
- Investigating accidents and categorizing them according to whether they were caused by systematic problems or the behavior of personnel
- Filing accident reports
- Conducting safety inspections and evaluate the results
- Managing a suggestion program and collecting ideas
- Initiating plans for the correction of safety problems
- Conducting safety meetings

Insurance

The CHFM is not expected to be an expert on insurance. However, the facility manager should be knowledgeable about the subject because he/she may be involved in selecting policies or filing claims for fire, fidelity, or liability insurance or for workers' compensation. For example, the CHFM must know what types of insurance are available and whether or not insurance against the risk of loss is cost effective. Top-level management should review insurance purchases and approve them, since there are serious drawbacks to both being overinsured and being underinsured. The facility manager may also be involved in any inspections or tours for insurance purposes.

CHFM Practice Test #1

Want to take this practice test in an online interactive format?
Check out the online resources page, which includes interactive practice questions and much more: **mometrix.com/resources719/chfm**

1. A hospital facility manager has been tasked to evaluate a surgical unit's compliance with rules and regulations concerning operating room fire exit drills. What is the minimum acceptable frequency the manager should consider compliant, and what NFPA standard should the manager reference to find the minimum acceptable frequency?

a. The minimum acceptable frequency is annually. The manager should reference the Health Care Facilities Code (NFPA 99).
b. The minimum acceptable frequency is annually. The manager should reference the Life Safety Code (NFPA 101).
c. The minimum acceptable frequency is quarterly. The manager should reference the Health Care Facilities Code (NFPA 99).
d. The minimum acceptable frequency is quarterly. The manager should reference the Life Safety Code (NFPA 101).

2. A facility's sprinkler system underwent an internal inspection in 2025. In what year should the system be reinspected to ensure compliance with NFPA 25?

a. 2026
b. 2028
c. 2030
d. 2035

3. A boiler is failing to reach adequate temperatures. Upon inspection, thick white deposits are discovered inside and determined to be the cause of the boiler's inadequacy. Which water quality should be addressed first to prevent this from occurring again?

a. pH
b. Hardness
c. Dissolved oxygen
d. Heat capacity

4. A health care facility manager has been tasked to do a financial analysis of a proposed lighting retrofit. The manager knows the following information concerning the financials of this project: utility peak demand charges are $12 per kW per month, the energy rate is $0.10 per kWh, peak demand will be reduced by 150 kW, energy savings are 500,000 kWh annually, and the project cost is $350,000. How many years will this project take to achieve a simple payback?

a. 3.98 years
b. 4.89 years
c. 5.21 years
d. 5.73 years

5. What is the best standard or guideline for energy simulation-aided design for hospitals, and at what stage of the design process should it be employed?

a. ASHRAE 170 is the best standard. It should be used in the final phase of design.
b. The FGI Guideline is the best guideline. It should be used in the design development phase.
c. ASHRAE 209 is the best standard. It should be used in the schematic design phase.
d. *Guide to Energy Management* is the best guideline. It should be employed in the schematic design phase.

6. Which of the following statements regarding egress width in different occupancies is correct?

a. Business occupancies and ambulatory health care (AHC) occupancies have the same egress width requirements.
b. Business occupancies have greater egress width requirements than ambulatory health care (AHC) occupancies.
c. Ambulatory health care (AHC) occupancies have greater egress width requirements than business occupancies
d. Egress width is the same for all occupancies.

7. A health care facility manager is concerned that a newly installed chiller may not meet peak demand during the hottest part of the summer. Which of the following documents should the manager evaluate to determine whether there is a system capacity shortfall?

a. HVAC equipment schedule
b. Functional performance test
c. Chiller operation and maintenance manual
d. American Society of Heating, Refrigerating, and Air Conditioning Engineers (ASHRAE) Handbook

8. An airborne isolation room has the following dimensions: 20 ft L, 20 ft W, 8 ft H. What is the least amount of air that can be supplied to provide the minimum required air changes per hour (ACH)?

a. 450 cubic feet per minute (cfm)
b. 510 cubic feet per minute (cfm)
c. 850 cubic feet per minute (cfm)
d. 640 cubic feet per minute (cfm)

9. The nurse manager of a dialysis unit has requested that maintenance staff perform water testing for the presence of residual disinfectant in the reverse osmosis (RO) water supplied to portable dialysis machines. Which of the following statements regarding this water test is correct?

a. The NFPA 99 risk category is 4, and a weekly test of total dissolved solids (TDS) should be performed
b. The NFPA 99 risk category is 1, and a daily test of total dissolved solids (TDS) should be performed.
c. The NFPA 99 risk category is 4, and a weekly test of total chlorine should be performed
d. The NFPA 99 risk category is 1, and a daily test of total chlorine should be performed.

10. A health care facility manager is conducting an annual review of Life Safety compliance in a three-story hospital using the International Building Code (IBC) as a standard. During the review, the manager notes the presence of a pipe chase that penetrates the first and second floors of the hospital. What fire-resistance rating for the pipe chase protective enclosure should the manager consider compliant with the IBC?

a. 30 minutes
b. 45 minutes
c. 1 hour
d. 2 hours

11. The greatest heat loss in a boiler is from the exiting flue gases. How does an economizer minimize these losses?

a. Economizers modulate combustion air to maximize fuel efficiency.
b. Economizers use a coil of water tubes in the flue gas outflow to scavenge heat from the hot gases of combustion and transfer that heat to the water in the boiler.
c. Economizers use a plate and frame heat exchanger to transfer heat from flue gas outflow and transfer that heat to combustion air.
d. Economizers use a tube bundle heat exchanger to scavenge heat from exiting flue gas and transfer that heat to a hydronic heating system.

12. Which of the following conditions does NOT describe legitimate grounds for a change order request?

a. Errors and omissions in construction documents
b. Unforeseen conditions
c. Phasing plans
d. Owner-requested changes to floor plans

13. Which of the following system components has the LOWEST priority for assessment and evaluation during a disaster drill designed to test the effectiveness of a hospital emergency power supply system (EPSS)?

a. Day tank float switch
b. Automatic transfer switch
c. Generator room emergency lights
d. Generator engine block heater

14. A health care facility manager has been tasked with determining which project, from a group of proposed projects, is the most profitable. If the proposed projects are mutually exclusive and have unequal lives and differing cash flows, then what is the best method of financial analysis?

a. Net present value (NPV)
b. Annual cost recovery
c. Cash flow diagram
d. Internal rate of return (IRR)

15. What organization enforces the public space provisions of the Americans with Disabilities Act (ADA)?

a. Equal Employment Opportunity Commission (EEOC)
b. United States Department of Justice (DOJ)
c. Occupational Safety and Health Administration (OSHA)
d. Facility Guidelines Institute (FGI)

16. A medical vacuum pump has been classified as a category 2 by NFPA 99 standards. Should this system fail, what potential risk can be expected?

a. There will likely be no impact on patient care.
b. The patient is likely to experience discomfort.
c. The patient and caregivers may experience minor injury.
d. The patient and caregivers may experience major injury or death.

17. What is the purpose of the ranking of deficiencies found during hazard surveillance rounds of hospital utility management systems?

a. The purpose is to improve the accuracy of root cause analyses of the most critical risks.
b. The purpose is to provide more funds for the resolution of critical deficiencies.
c. The purpose is to reduce the total number of deficiencies.
d. The purpose is to enable managers to focus on fixing the most critical deficiencies first.

18. A health care facility manager is evaluating project schedule effects caused by a delay in the delivery of an air handling unit for a new medical-surgical unit. Which of the following scenarios provides the greatest likelihood for completing the project on time?

a. The installation of the air handling unit is on the critical path, and the project uses phased occupancy.
b. The installation of the air handling unit was not on the critical path, and the project used phased occupancy.
c. The installation of the air handling unit was on the critical path, and the project did not use phased occupancy.
d. The installation of the air handling unit was not on the critical path, and the project did not use phased occupancy.

19. If a hospital maintenance department manager has budgeted labor at 10% of the total department budget, the total department budget is $1,000,000, and actual labor expenditures are $125,000, then what is the percent of actual labor variance from the amount budgeted for labor?

a. The actual labor exceeds the budgeted overtime by 25%.
b. The actual overtime is 75% of the budgeted overtime.
c. The actual overtime budget exceeds the budgeted overtime by 20%.
d. The actual overtime budget is 80% of the budgeted overtime.

20. Frequently, when hospital facility managers are working on regulatory issues, they must refer to NFPA codes for the specific details of compliance. Given that there are multiple editions of each NFPA code, how do hospital facility managers know which edition of an NFPA code is the one that should be referenced?

a. The Center for Medicare & Medicaid Services (CMS) automatically accepts the most recent edition of the Life Safety Code (NFPA 101) on its publication date, and facility managers know that Referenced Publications (Chapter 2) of the most recent edition of NFPA 101 specifies which editions of other NFPA codes should be referenced in order to comply with NFPA 101.
b. The Center for Medicare & Medicaid Services (CMS) has adopted the 2012 edition of The Life Safety Code (NFPA 101), and facility managers know that Referenced Publications (Chapter 2) of the 2012 edition of NFPA 101 specifies which editions of other NFPA codes should be referenced in order to comply with the 2012 edition of NFPA 101.
c. The Center for Medicare & Medicaid Services (CMS) has adopted the 2012 edition of the Health Care Facilities Code (NFPA 99), and facility managers know that Referenced Publications (Chapter 2) of the 2012 edition of NFPA 99 specifies which editions of other NFPA codes should be referenced in order to comply with the 2012 edition of NFPA 99.
d. The Center for Medicare & Medicaid Services (CMS) automatically accepts the most recent edition of the Health Care Facilities Code (NFPA 99) on its publication date, and facility managers know that Referenced Publications (Chapter 2) of the most recent edition of NFPA 99 specifies which editions of other NFPA codes should be referenced in order to comply with the NFPA 99.

21. Many hospitals exist in areas that are prone to earthquakes. These healthcare facilities must be designed to provide safety for patients in the event of a major earthquake. Post-earthquake fires fueled by natural gas leaks from ruptured lines are one of the greatest risks to hospital patients during these emergencies. How can healthcare facility managers mitigate this risk?

a. Healthcare facility managers mitigate this risk by installing isolation valves at the natural gas utility service entrance meter station.
b. Healthcare facility managers mitigate this risk by installing seismic valves at the natural gas utility service entrance meter station.
c. Healthcare facility managers mitigate this risk by installing bypass valves at the natural gas utility service entrance meter station.
d. Healthcare facility managers mitigate this risk by installing pressure regulating valves at the natural gas utility service entrance meter station.

22. A health care facility manager has been assigned to oversee the field acceptance of a new fire pump. The manager's first order of business is deciding who needs to be present. What code should the manager reference, and who is required by this code to be present for the field acceptance tests?

a. A representative of the local fire department is required to be present to witness the tests. This requirement can be found in the Standard for Inspection, Testing, and Maintenance of Water-Based Fire Protection Systems (NFPA 25).
b. A representative of the local fire department is required to be present to witness the tests. This requirement can be found in the Standard for Installation of Stationary Pumps for Fire Protection (NFPA 20).
c. All the fire pump major component manufacturers (or their factory-authorized representatives) are required to be present to witness the tests. This requirement can be found in the Standard for Inspection, Testing, and Maintenance of Water-Based Fire Protection Systems (NFPA 25).
d. All the fire pump major component manufacturers (or their factory-authorized representatives) are required to be present to witness the tests. This requirement can be found in the Standard for Installation of Stationary Pumps for Fire Protection (NFPA 20).

23. Which of the following statements concerning confined space entry is NOT correct?

a. Employees making permit space rescues must practice permit space rescue at least once every 12 months.
b. Confined space entry attendants may not enter the confined space to attempt a rescue.
c. At least one member of a confined space rescue team must be certified in first aid.
d. Confined space entry attendants must be aware of the behavioral effects entrants to the space would display if exposed to a hazard.

24. Which of the following strategies would be most effective as a corrective action for a feeder circuit with a power factor of 0.72?

a. Rebalance the electrical loads supplied by the feeder.
b. Connect an inductor to the feeder load.
c. Connect a capacitor to the feeder load.
d. Reduce the electrical load on the feeder.

25. Although there is no requirement for Legionella testing, a health care organization may include Legionella testing as part of the waterborne pathogen management plan. If an organization's plan calls for Legionella testing in the absence of suspected or confirmed facility-associated disease, what does the American Society of Heating, Refrigerating, and Air Conditioning Engineers (ASHRAE) recommend regarding the selection of a testing laboratory?

a. Use a laboratory that turns samples around in 72 hours or less.
b. Use a laboratory that is certified to be proficient and accredited to perform Legionella testing by a recognized accrediting organization.
c. Use a laboratory that can identify the serogroup of any positive Legionella test results.
d. Use a laboratory that can perform heterotrophic plate counts at points of use that test positive for Legionella.

26. What is the maximum permitted travel distance to an exit access door on an inpatient sleeping suite protected by an automatic sprinkler system? Assume this health care occupancy is classified as existing construction.

a. 75 feet
b. 100 feet
c. 150 feet
d. 200 feet

27. A hospital has installed a new emergency generator and is developing preventative maintenance (PM) tasks. What NFPA standard should be referenced when determining minimum testing intervals?

a. NFPA 110
b. NFPA 101
c. NFPA 70
d. NFPA 37

28. A health care facility manager wants to eliminate brief power interruptions caused by unexpectedly switching from normal power to emergency power. Which of the following options would be most effective in achieving this?

a. Stored emergency power supply system (SEPSS)
b. Closed transition automatic transfer switch (ATS)
c. Uninterruptible power system (UPS)
d. Ground fault circuit interrupter (GFCI)

29. Which of the following health care project management tools is effective in reducing issues such as intertrade, above-ceiling "turf" clashes?

a. Building Information Modeling (BIM)
b. Pre-construction risk assessment (PCRA)
c. Critical Path Method (CPM)
d. Interim Life Safety Measures (ILSM)

30. With respect to continuity of critical patient care, what planning tasks should most concern a health care facility manager preparing for a critical care area switchgear replacement project?

a. Validation of the one-line diagram of the health care facility emergency power supply system (EPSS) and identification of single points of failure
b. Determination of appropriate Interim Life Safety Measures (ILSM) and development of an infection control risk mitigation (ICRA) plan
c. Infrared (IR) imaging of the switchgear
d. Completion of a test and balance (TAB) survey

31. A health care facility manager is troubleshooting a rooftop air conditioner that is short cycling (i.e., experiencing shorter refrigeration cycles). Which of the following conditions is least likely to cause short cycling?

a. Dirty air filters
b. Dirty evaporator coil
c. Clogged condensate drain line
d. Low refrigerant level

32. Which of the following bonds best protects subcontractors from financial loss?

a. Surety bond
b. Performance bond
c. Payment bond
d. Bid bond

33. During the building tour session of a mock Joint Commission Physical Environment survey, a health care facility manager observes that the diesel fuel tank serving the fire pump diesel engine is half full. Is this fuel level compliant with regulatory requirements, and what NFPA standard governs this?

a. Yes, it is compliant. The Standard for the Inspection, Testing, and Maintenance of Water-Based Fire Protection Systems (NFPA 25) requires that "the fuel tank is at least 1/2 full."
b. No, it is not compliant. The Standard for the Inspection, Testing, and Maintenance of Stationary Fire Pumps (NFPA 20) requires that "the fuel tank is over 1/2 full."
c. Yes, it is compliant. The Standard for the Inspection, Testing, and Maintenance of Stationary Fire Pumps (NFPA 20) requires that "the fuel tank is at least 1/3 full."
d. No, it is not compliant. The Standard for the Inspection, Testing, and Maintenance of Water-Based Fire Protection Systems (NFPA 25) requires that "the fuel tank is at least 2/3 full."

34. A facility's main switchgear has been identified as Condition 3 per NFPA standards. How often should infrared thermography be performed on this equipment?

a. Every 4 months
b. Every 6 months
c. Every 12 months
d. Every 24 months

35. Airborne infection isolation rooms (AIIRs) are being built in a facility's new wing. How many air changes per hour are required within these rooms?

a. 4
b. 6
c. 8
d. 12

36. What standard governs the upkeep of engine-driven fire pumps that serve hospitals?

a. The Life Safety Code (NFPA 101)
b. The Standard for the Installation of Stationary Pumps for Fire Protection (NFPA 20)
c. The Standard for the Installation and Use of Stationary Combustion Engines (NFPA 37)
d. The Standard for the Inspection, Testing, and Maintenance of Water-Based Fire Protection Systems (NFPA 25)

37. A health care facility manager has been tasked to design a Life Safety compliance checklist for hazard surveillance rounding of a medical-surgical patient care unit constructed in 2021. Which of the choices below is the best checklist item narrative for validating compliance with the Life Safety Code (LSC) (NFPA 101) requirements for the unobstructed clear width of a corridor?

a. Is the unobstructed clear corridor width less than eight feet?
b. Is the unobstructed clear corridor width less than six feet?
c. Is the unobstructed clear corridor width less than five feet?
d. Is the unobstructed clear corridor width less than four feet?

38. Which of the following statements regarding hospital medical gas equipment is correct?

a. There are three risk categories for hospital medical gas equipment established by the Health Care Facilities Code (NFPA 99). Category 3 is used to classify hospital medical gas equipment with the highest risk to patients and staff.
b. There are four risk categories for hospital medical gas equipment established by the Health Care Facilities Code (NFPA 99). Category 1 is used to classify hospital medical gas equipment with the highest risk to patients and staff.
c. There are three risk categories for hospital medical gas equipment established by the Life Safety Code (NFPA 101). Category 1 is used to classify hospital medical gas equipment with the highest risk to patients and staff.
d. There are four risk categories for hospital medical gas equipment established by the Life Safety Code (NFPA 101). Category 4 is used to classify hospital medical gas equipment with the highest risk to patients and staff.

39. A hospital facility manager has been tasked to review a hospital contractor's compliance with applicable health and safety regulations governing asbestos removal. What reference should the manager consult to determine compliance?

a. EPA Title 40 CFR
b. DOT Title 49 CFR
c. OSHA Title 29 CFR
d. NIOSH Title 29 CFR

40. Which of the following statements is correct?

a. The FCI drives the operational budget.
b. The FCI drives the utility budget.
c. The FCI drives the safety budget.
d. The FCI drives the capital budget.

41. How is the safety of high-pressure steam boilers assured by hospital facility management practices?

a. The safety of high-pressure boilers is assured by scheduling boiler licensing inspections every five years, tearing down all boilers for internal inspection, and correcting any deficiencies noted by the boiler inspector prior to returning the boilers to service.
b. The safety of high-pressure boilers is assured by scheduling annual boiler licensing inspections, tearing down any boilers requested to be internally inspected by the boiler inspector, allowing the boiler inspector to inspect the boilers, and correcting any deficiencies noted by the boiler inspector prior to returning the boilers to service.
c. The safety of high-pressure boilers is assured by scheduling hydrostatic testing of the pressure vessel every year, correcting any deficiencies noted during the test, and re-testing to confirm effective repair.
d. The safety of high-pressure boilers is assured by completing annual safety valve replacement and maintaining the presence of a state-licensed boiler operator anytime boilers operate.

42. The addition and subsequent operation of a new chiller raises a hospital's energy use intensity from 80 per kBtu per square foot to 95 kBtu per square foot. If the hospital has an area of 1.5 million square feet and energy costs are $0.012 per kBtu, then what energy cost increase should the hospital expect?

a. $230,000 per year
b. $250,000 per year
c. $260,000 per year
d. $270,000 per year

43. If hospital main entrances employ electrically powered sliding automatic doors, then how do hospital facility managers ensure facility occupants can exit if there is a fire during an electrical power failure?

a. Hospital facility managers ensure operability of electrically powered sliding glass doors during power failures by regular inspection, testing, and maintenance (ITM) of the door operator backup battery power supply system.
b. Hospital facility managers ensure operability of electrically powered sliding glass doors during power failures by ensuring regular inspection, testing, and maintenance (ITM) of the emergency "push to open" function of each of the leaves of a sliding door system.
c. Hospital facility managers ensure operability of electrically powered sliding glass doors during power failures by regular inspection, testing, and maintenance (ITM) of the automatic transfer switch (ATS) that provides backup electrical power during utility failures.
d. Hospital facility managers ensure operability of electrically powered sliding glass doors during power failures by regular inspection, testing, and maintenance (ITM) of the "open on failure" function of the door control sequencing system.

44. While updating a project schedule, a health care facility manager notes that a critical task has only two immediate successor tasks. The manager also notes that these two tasks are to be executed concurrently, and they have different durations. Task X has a duration of 5 days, and task Y has a duration of 10 days. The health care facility manager has been informed that the duration of task X must be tripled due to an unresolvable issue. After the manager makes the schedule update, which of these tasks is on the critical path, and how much float time is generated for which task?

a. Both tasks are on the critical path, and no float time is generated.
b. Task X is on the critical path, and five days of float time is generated for task Y.
c. Task Y is on the critical path and has five days of float time.
d. Task X is on the critical path, and there is no float time.

45. One approach a hospital facility manager may use to mitigate the harmful effects of smoke from wildfires is replacement of existing air filters with higher efficiency air filters. What must be known before using this approach?

a. The air handling unit air supply volume in cubic feet per minute (CFM)
b. The ability of the fan motors to move air through the new filters
c. Air changes per hour in patient sleeping rooms
d. The percent of supply air that is fresh outside air (not recirculated)

46. Management receives a proposal with an escalation clause tied to annual increases of Consumer Price Index – Urban (CPI-U) plus 2%. CPI-U averages 4%. What compounded percentage increase will occur over 3 years?

a. 17.6%
b. 19.1%
c. 22.7%
d. 23.8%

47. A facility is located in a coastal area that is prone to frequent storms characterized by strong winds and heavy rains. What standard is the most crucial in protecting windows from associated damage?

a. ASTM E1996
b. ASTM E84
c. ASTM E1300
d. ASTM E8

48. A health care facility manager has secured a vendor to validate the health care organization's existing Life Safety drawings. Which of the following documents would be most useful to the vendor during the facility tour?

a. Suppression system hydraulic calculations
b. Health care facility evacuation diagrams
c. As-built drawings
d. Certificates of occupancy

49. A hospital facility manager has been asked to evaluate a hyperbaric treatment center's compliance with rules and regulations concerning fire drills. What two important points should the manager check to assess compliance?

a. The manager should check to make sure that fire drills are conducted quarterly and that fire drill documentation includes a measurement of the time required to evacuate a single patient.
b. The manager should check to make sure that fire drills are conducted annually and that fire drill documentation includes a measurement of the time required to evacuate a single patient.
c. The manager should check to make sure that fire drills are conducted annually and that fire drill documentation includes a measurement of the time required to evacuate a full complement of patients.
d. The manager should check to make sure that fire drills are conducted quarterly and that fire drill documentation includes a measurement of the time required to evacuate a full complement of patients.

50. Which of the following construction project activities is most affected by delayed subcontractor drawings?

a. HVAC test and balance
b. Pressure testing of domestic hot and cold water
c. Mechanical, electrical, and plumbing (MEP) coordination
d. Value engineering

51. Suppose a hospital pays an hourly maintenance technician every two weeks. Further, suppose the technician has worked 46 hours in week 1 and 43 hours in week 2 of the current pay period. How should the technician's overtime pay for this pay period be calculated?

a. Add the weekly totals and divide by two to get the average hours per week over the pay period. Any hours over 40 in either week must be paid as overtime.
b. Total each week's hours separately. Pay for any hours over 40 in either week as overtime.
c. Any hours worked over 80 in a two-week pay period should be paid at the overtime rate.
d. Only pay the technician overtime for the days the technician worked more than 8 hours.

52. A hospital facility manager has been tasked to review construction drawings for compliance with the 1991 Americans with Disabilities Act (ADA). During the review, the manager notes that the plans specify a front-approach counter in the lobby that is 38 inches above the finished floor (AFF) and a parallel-approach counter at the outpatient pharmacy that is 36 inches AFF. What should the manager report concerning these counters?

a. The manager should report that neither counter is compliant with the Americans with Disabilities Act (ADA).
b. The manager should report that the height of the front-approach counter is compliant with the Americans with Disabilities Act (ADA), and the height of the parallel-approach counter is not compliant.
c. The manager should report that both counters are compliant with the Americans with Disabilities Act (ADA).
d. The manager should report that the height of the front-approach counter is not compliant with the Americans with Disabilities Act (ADA), and the height of the parallel-approach counter is compliant.

53. A health care facility manager troubleshoots an electrical fault using the facility's current as-built one-line electrical diagram as a reference. The manager determines that the area of the fault is represented by a dashed conduit line on the diagram. What does the dashed conduit line most likely represent?

a. Mechanically linked conduit bodies
b. Alternate feed to an automatic transfer switch
c. Hidden electrical conduit
d. Existing conduit that is to be removed

54. Where would a hospital facility manager find the ventilation requirements for the design of airborne isolation patient sleeping rooms?

a. The ventilation requirements for the design of airborne isolation patient sleeping rooms are provided in ASHRAE 170-2017. ASHRAE 170-2017 has been incorporated into the Health Care Facilities Code (NFPA 99).
b. The ventilation requirements for the design of airborne isolation patient sleeping rooms are provided in ASHRAE 170-2017. ASHRAE 170-2017 has been incorporated into the Facility Guidelines Institute (FGI) Guidelines publication.
c. The ventilation requirements for the design of airborne isolation patient sleeping rooms are provided in ASHRAE 90.1. ASHRAE 90.1 has been incorporated into the Facility Guidelines Institute (FGI) Guidelines publication
d. The ventilation requirements for the design of airborne isolation patient sleeping rooms are provided in ASHRAE 90.1. ASHRAE 90.1 has been incorporated into the Health Care Facilities Code (NFPA 99).

55. A hospital facility manager is planning the four-hour generator load test that is required every 36 months. What are two important components of executing this test?

a. An alternate generator must be provided by the organization, and it must be tested in accordance with NFPA 110.
b. The test must be conducted continuously, and the load must be at least 30% of the nameplate rating.
c. The generator fuel quality must be tested, and it must be tested in accordance with an ASTM standard.
d. The test must employ a load bank, and the power factor used to calculate load current must be 1.0.

56. A hospital facility manager is seeking Federal Emergency Management Agency (FEMA) funds to pay for the mitigation of hurricane damage to hospital buildings and equipment. Under which FEMA mitigation category is the manager's health care organization eligible to apply?

a. Category F
b. Category E
c. Category B
d. Category C

57. How often should hospital maintenance staff be trained in Lockout/Tagout procedures in order for a health care organization to be considered compliant with OSHA regulations?

a. During orientation and monthly thereafter
b. During orientation and quarterly thereafter
c. During orientation and semiannually thereafter
d. During orientation and annually thereafter

58. A hospital facility manager is conducting a financial analysis of a proposed photovoltaic (PV) array project and wishes to calculate the annual energy cost avoidance. Given that the PV array will generate 1.2 GWh per year, the utility supply charge is $0.10 per kWh, the delivery charge is $0.07 per kWh, the blended rate is $0.20 per kWh, and the annual energy usage is 3.6 GWh, what is the annual energy cost avoidance of this PV array project?

a. $220,000
b. $240,000
c. $260,000
d. $280,000

59. A hospital facility manager is determining whether a construction project that will add square feet to the hospital footprint is necessary. If the manager uses the Strengths, Weaknesses, Opportunities, and Threats (SWOT) analysis technique, then how would the project's future effect on Medicare reimbursement to the hospital be assessed?

a. The project's future effect on Medicare reimbursement to the hospital could be considered either an Opportunity or a Threat, depending on whether reimbursement increases or decreases due to project execution.
b. The project's future effect on Medicare reimbursement to the hospital could be considered either a Strength or a Weakness, depending on whether reimbursement increases or decreases due to project execution.
c. The project's future effect on Medicare reimbursement to the hospital could be considered either an Opportunity or a Weakness, depending on whether reimbursement increases or decreases due to project execution.
d. The project's future effect on Medicare reimbursement to the hospital could be considered either a Strength or a Threat, depending on whether reimbursement increases or decreases due to project execution.

60. A boiler dry burn event occurs when a boiler system continues to fire despite a failure of the boiler makeup water supply system to keep water in the boiler pressure vessel. Which of the following events do NOT add to the likelihood of a boiler dry burn event?

a. Human error
b. Alarm failure
c. Fuel pump failure
d. Boiler makeup water pump failure

61. How should health care organizations document National Fire Protection Association (NFPA) compliance with the requirements for monthly load tests of their emergency power supply systems (EPSS)?

a. Health care organizations should document monthly load tests of their emergency power supply systems (EPSS) on the EPSS Operation and Testing Log found in Chapter 6 (Electrical Systems) of the Health Care Facilities Code (NFPA 99).
b. Health care organizations should document monthly load tests of their emergency power supply systems (EPSS) on the EPSS Operation and Testing Log found in Annex A (Explanatory Information) of the Standard for Emergency and Standby Power Systems (NFPA 110).
c. Health care organizations should document monthly load tests of their emergency power supply systems (EPSS) in accordance with the Health Care Facilities Code (NFPA 99) Chapter 6 (Electrical Systems), paragraph 6.4.4.2 (Record Keeping).
d. Health care organizations should document monthly load tests of their EPSS in accordance with the Standard for Emergency and Standby Power Systems (NFPA 110), Chapter 8 (Routine Maintenance and Operational Testing), paragraph 8.3.4.1 (Permanent Record).

62. How does a simple payback period differ from a discounted payback period?

a. Discounted payback periods consider depreciation. Simple payback periods do not.
b. A simple payback period uses the same interest rate for each alternative. Discounted payback periods do not.
c. Discounted payback periods consider taxes. Simple payback periods do not.
d. Discounted payback periods consider the time value of money as an expense. Simple payback periods do not.

63. What function does an MRI quench vent perform, and what risk does it mitigate?

a. The quench vent exhausts liquid helium to atmospheric pressure at a safe location outside the building. It mitigates magnetic field collapse risks that the MRI uses for imaging patients.
b. The quench vent exhausts liquid nitrogen to atmospheric pressure at a safe location outside the building. It mitigates the asphyxiation risk to building occupants due to oxygen displacement by nitrogen gas.
c. The quench vent exhausts liquid helium to atmospheric pressure at a safe location outside the building. It mitigates the asphyxiation risk to building occupants due to oxygen displacement by helium gas.
d. The quench vent exhausts liquid nitrogen to atmospheric pressure at a safe location outside the building. It mitigates magnetic field collapse risks that the MRI uses for imaging patients.

64. If a health care facility manager wants to reduce the buildup of scale on the interior surfaces of steam boilers, then the manager should do which of the following?

a. Minimize boiler water total dissolved solids (TDS).
b. Maximize boiler water total dissolved solids (TDS).
c. Oxygenate the boiler water.
d. Lower the pH of the boiler feedwater.

65. What category of hospital heliports serves helicopters less than 15 meters in overall length?

a. H-1
b. H-2
c. H-3
d. H-4

66. Submission of a final pay application requires which of the following two closeout tasks be completed before submission?

a. Punch list completion and delivery of operation and maintenance manuals
b. HVAC commissioning and hydrostatic testing
c. Soil analysis and geotechnical surveys
d. Certificate of Occupancy (CO) and medical gas testing for cross connections

67. The manager of an acute care facility wants to compare the facility's Energy Use Intensity (EUI) percentile to that of peer facilities. What database should be referenced?

a. The CMS Hospital Quality Initiative Public Reports
b. The Joint Commission Accreditation Database
c. The EPA Energy Star Portfolio Manager
d. The American Hospital Association Annual Survey Database

68. A health care facility manager wishes to determine whether the lease or purchase of an asset is more profitable. What method of financial analysis should the manager use to make this determination?

a. Net present value (NPV) analysis
b. Annual cost method of analysis
c. Simple payback analysis
d. Straight-line depreciation analysis

69. Which of the following statements about a hospital's essential electrical system (EES) is correct?

a. The Health Care Facilities Code (NFPA 99) definition says an essential electrical system (EES) consists of alternate power sources and all connected electrical distribution systems. NFPA 99 further defines an EES as purpose-built to do two things: provide continuity of electric power and minimize disruption within the internal wiring system.
b. The Health Care Facilities Code (NFPA 99) says an essential electrical system (EES) consists of a generator (or bank of generators) and all connected electrical distribution panels and subpanels. NFPA 99 also says an EES is purpose-built to do two things: provide continuity of electrical power and minimize disruption within the external wiring system.
c. The National Electrical Code (NEC) (NFPA 70) says an essential electrical system (EES) consists of alternate power sources and all connected electrical distribution systems. NFPA 70 also says an EES is purpose-built to do two things: provide continuity of electrical power and minimize power losses within the internal wiring system.
d. The National Electrical Code (NEC) (NFPA 70) says an essential electrical system (EES) consists of a generator (or bank of generators) and all connected electrical distribution panels and subpanels. NFPA 70 also says an EES is purpose-built to do two things: provide continuity of electrical power and minimize disruption within the external wiring system.

70. Which of the following key performance indicators (KPIs) best measures the effectiveness of a health care organization's planning for a construction project?

a. Cost variance from budget and schedule variance from on-time completion
b. Sustainability indexes and energy benchmarks
c. Construction safety protocols and safety audit checklists
d. Energy Use Intensity (EUI) of the new occupied space

71. What are the OSHA requirements for the documentation of job hazard assessments?

a. There must be a typed document that identifies the workplace assessed, the person assessing, and the date assessed. The document must also specifically self-identify as a job hazard assessment.
b. There must be a written document that certifies the workplace assessed, the person certifying the assessment, and the date assessed. The document must also specifically self-identify as an assessment certification.
c. There must be a written document that identifies the workplace assessed, the person assessing, and the date assessed. The document must also specifically list what was assessed and the method of assessment.
d. There must be a typed document that certifies the workplace assessed, the person certifying the assessment, and the date assessed. The document must also specifically list what was assessed and the method of assessment.

72. A hospital has accumulated waste in the form of discarded lamps and batteries. Which of the following statements is true regarding this waste?

a. The discarded lamps and batteries should be classified as Hazardous Waste and may be accumulated for up to one year.
b. The discarded lamps and batteries should be classified as Universal Waste and may be accumulated for up to one year.
c. The discarded lamps and batteries should be classified as Hazardous Waste and may be accumulated for up to six months.
d. The discarded lamps and batteries should be classified as Universal Waste and may be accumulated for up to six months.

73. Which of the following project management tools is used to track the resolution of minor construction defects, and at what stage of the project is it to be used?

a. A Certificate of Substantial Completion is used prior to project closeout.
b. A punch list is used during project closeout.
c. A field observation report is used during project closeout.
d. A warranty log is used for the construction phase.

74. Which of the following scenarios is a plausible sequence of events resulting in an unplanned loss of chilled water for air conditioning in an operating room?

a. A maintenance technician turns off a cooling tower makeup water valve prior to repairing a minor leak. Later, the cooling tower low water cutoff engages and shuts down the cooling tower. Consequently, the chiller refrigerant temperature rises because there is no cooling tower water to cool it. Because chiller refrigerant pressure rises with temperature, the refrigerant high-pressure lockout threshold is reached, and the chiller is locked out due to high refrigerant pressure.
b. A maintenance technician turns off the circuit breaker for an air handling unit supply fan prior to changing the filters for that unit. Consequently, the chilled water temperature in the water circulating through the air handling unit fan coil drops. Later, the fan coil low temperature cutoff engages and shuts down the chilled water circulating pumps.
c. A maintenance technician turns off an air handling unit supply fan to replace the UV lamps used to irradiate the fan coil. Consequently, the air handling unit static pressure drops and trips the static pressure low limit relay. This relay is interlocked with the cooling tower water circulating pump, so the pump shuts down. The centrifugal chiller refrigerant temperature rises because there is no cooling tower water to cool it. The chiller refrigerant pressure rises with temperature. The high-pressure lockout threshold is reached, and the chiller is locked out due to high pressure.
d. A maintenance technician turns off an air handling unit to test the fire alarm relay. After, the air handling unit will not restart due to the failure of an end switch on the outside air damper. The end switch is interlocked with the cooling tower, so the tower shuts down. The chiller refrigerant temperature rises because there is no cooling tower to cool it. The chiller refrigerant pressure rises with the temperature, so the high-pressure lockout threshold is reached, and the chiller is locked out due to high pressure.

75. A hospital facility manager has been tasked to review a service contract for inspection, testing, and maintenance (ITM) of the hospital's fire alarm, notification, and detection systems. Which of the following contract indemnification arrangements is best for the hospital?

a. The hospital indemnifies the vendor from loss with an insurance policy.
b. The vendor and the hospital mutually indemnify each other from loss with an insurance policy.
c. The service vendor indemnifies the hospital from loss with an insurance policy.
d. Neither party should indemnify the other.

76. Under what circumstances would a variable frequency drive (VFD) be a better choice than a premium efficiency motor?

a. A variable frequency drive (VFD) is a better choice when there is a low power factor.
b. A variable frequency drive (VFD) is a better choice when the ambient temperature is high.
c. A variable frequency drive (VFD) is a better choice when the load is static.
d. A variable frequency drive (VFD) is a better choice when the load is dynamic.

77. A hospital facility manager has been tasked to create a standard operating procedure for the annual certification of underground storage tanks (USTs). What regulatory agency should the procedure document as the certifier of underground storage tanks?

a. Occupational Safety and Health Administration (OSHA)
b. Environmental Protection Agency (EPA)
c. The federally designated agency
d. The state-designated agency

78. Which of the following test methods is best for verifying proper pressurization of air in a protective environment (PE) room, and what should that pressurization be?

a. The best way to verify proper pressurization of a protective environment (PE) room is to use a swing vane anemometer to measure differential pressure. PE rooms should be positively pressurized
b. The best way to verify proper pressurization of a protective environment (PE) room is to use a manometer that measures differential pressure. PE rooms should be positively pressurized.
c. The best way to verify proper pressurization of a protective environment (PE) room is to use a swing vane anemometer to measure differential pressure. PE rooms should be negatively pressurized.
d. The best way to verify proper pressurization of a protective environment (PE) room is to use a manometer that measures differential pressure. PE rooms should be negatively pressurized.

79. A hospital facility manager reviewing deficiencies listed in an energy management report for the facility's electrical distribution system notes that one feeder has a power factor of 0.72. Which corrective course of action is best?

a. Install a capacitor bank at the feeder to increase the power factor.
b. Install a capacitor bank at the electrical service entrance to increase the power factor.
c. Install an inductor bank at the feeder to increase the power factor.
d. Install an inductor bank at the electrical service entrance to increase the power factor.

80. A hospital facility manager is conducting a code review for an upcoming renovation project and discovers a local building code that conflicts with the Life Safety Code (LSC). How can the manager resolve this discrepancy?

a. Apply to CMS for a waiver of the specific local code that conflicts with the LSC.
b. Develop a compliance strategy that complies with the most stringent of the codes in conflict.
c. The LSC takes precedence over local regulations, so the manager should comply with the LSC.
d. Local regulations supersede all others, so the manager should comply with the local code.

81. A hospital facility manager notes a trip hazard due to a cracked sidewalk at the employee entrance from the hospital parking lot. What CMS K-Tag applies to this deficiency?

a. K42: Grounds and Equipment
b. K211: Means of Egress
c. K761: Maintenance, Inspection, and Testing
d. K900: Other

82. Where would a health care facility manager expect to find waste gas scavenging equipment?

a. Boiler room
b. Operating room
c. Elevator machine room
d. MRI machine room

83. A health care organization wishes to deviate from recommended medical equipment maintenance practices. Which of the following statements is true regarding an organization's ability to deviate from recommendations?

a. A health care organization may deviate from recommendations if it is planning to design more efficient and effective medical equipment maintenance activities that do not reduce patient safety, and the Food and Drug Administration (FDA) permits an Alternative Equipment Maintenance (AEM) program.
b. A health care organization may deviate from recommendations if it has learned through experience of more efficient and effective maintenance activities that do not reduce the safety of the equipment, and the Centers for Medicare & Medicaid Services (CMS) facilitates this by permitting an Alternate Equipment Maintenance (AEM) program.
c. A health care organization may deviate from recommendations if it has learned through experience of more efficient and effective maintenance activities that do not reduce patient safety, and the National Institutes of Health (NIH) facilitates this by permitting a Reliability Centered Maintenance (RCM) program.
d. A health care organization may deviate from recommendations if it is planning to design more efficient and effective medical equipment maintenance activities that do not reduce the safety of the equipment, and the American Society for Health Care Engineering (ASHE) facilitates this by permitting Reliability-Centered Maintenance (RCM).

84. Which process reduces project lender risk when a funding draw is requested?

a. The surety process reduces lender risk.
b. The lien waiver process reduces lender risk.
c. The subcontractor vetting process reduces lender risk.
d. The performance bond process reduces lender risk.

85. Which protocol is used by energy service companies (ESCOs) to verify savings?

a. Building Automation and Control Networks (BACnet)
b. Transmission Control Protocol/Internet Protocol (TCP/IP)
c. International Performance Measurement and Verification Protocol (IPMVP)
d. International Electrotechnical Commission (IEC) 62056

86. What is the most frequent inspection, testing, and maintenance (ITM) interval required for hospital elevators?

a. The most frequent hospital elevator ITM interval is weekly testing of firefighters' emergency operation.
b. The most frequent hospital elevator ITM interval is monthly testing of firefighters' emergency operation.
c. The most frequent hospital elevator ITM interval is a quarterly check of firefighters' emergency operation.
d. The most frequent hospital elevator ITM interval is annual testing of firefighters' emergency operation.

87. What does an energy control program refer to for a hospital facility manager?

a. EPA software used to track Energy Star ratings
b. Direct digital control (DDC) software for HVAC
c. Building management system (BMS) program
d. Lockout/Tagout program

88. A hospital facility manager has been asked to determine how a change in chiller performance will affect the facility's energy budget. If the chiller performance is changing from 0.65 [kW/ton] to 0.9 [kW/ton], then what will the budgetary effects be?

a. A rise in energy costs due to an increase of 38.5% in chiller energy consumption.
b. A drop in energy costs due to a decrease of 38.5% in chiller energy consumption.
c. A rise in energy costs due to an increase of 27.7% in chiller energy consumption.
d. A drop in energy costs due to an increase of 27.7% in chiller energy consumption.

89. Most health care facilities use acronyms to help staff recall emergency procedures. What is an emergency procedure acronym commonly used by staff to recall emergency actions for response to a fire?

a. RACE: rescue, activate fire alarm, close doors, evacuate
b. SAFE: save victims, activate fire alarm, evacuate
c. PASS: pull the pin, aim the nozzle, squeeze the handle, sweep the nozzle from side to side while aiming for the base of the flame
d. CALL: contact fire department, activate alarm, look for victims, leave the area

90. What are the construction-related NFPA regulatory code triggers in a health care occupancy that require adjacent areas to be brought up to code?

a. If an area to be renovated has no smoke detection, then a sprinkler system must be installed in any adjacent area.
b. If an area of renovation is more than 50% of the area of a smoke compartment or greater than 4,500 square feet, then adjacent areas must be brought up to code.
c. If the Local Authority Having Jurisdiction (LAHJ) notifies the Architect of Record of Life Safety deficiencies, then areas adjacent to these deficiencies must be brought up to code.
d. If the date of the approved plans predates current editions of NFPA codes, then adjacent areas must be upgraded.

91. A hospital facility manager is supervising a mold remediation project in a surgical suite. Once the project is completed, how will the manager know if it is safe to reopen the operating rooms?

a. The manager will arrange for air and surface sampling for each operating room.
b. The manager will measure and record temperature and relative humidity for each operating room to confirm no deviations from ASHRAE 170 requirements.
c. The manager will engage the services of a test and balance (TAB) technician to confirm the HVAC system is providing the required air changes per hour (ACH) and proper pressurization for each operating room.
d. The manager will arrange for the measurement of air particulate concentration for each operating room.

92. The leadership of a health care organization has tasked a hospital facility manager to create a facility-specific Spill Prevention, Control, and Countermeasure (SPCC) plan for a hospital. Which of the following statements best describes how the facility manager should prepare this plan?

a. The facility manager should include community Right-to-Know information and worker emergency response information, as documented in Title 29 CFR Part 1910.
b. The facility manager should include emergency response procedures and facility oil storage information, as documented in Title 40 CFR. Part 112
c. The facility manager should include community Right-to-Know information and facility oil storage information, as documented in the Superfund Amendments and Reauthorization Act (SARA), Title III.
d. The facility manager should include local emergency response procedures and facility HAZMAT information, as documented in the facility-specific master plans of the Local Emergency Planning Committee (LEPC).

93. Hospital facility managers routinely review records of inspection, testing, and maintenance (ITM). During one such review, a health care facility manager noted the following completion dates for the following instances of ITM. Which of these instances should most concern the manager?

a. Fire damper inspection, testing, and maintenance (ITM): Last completed 5 years and 6 months before the date of the review by the hospital facility manager
b. Dry system sprinkler gauge inspections: Last completed 26 days before the date of the review by the hospital facility manager
c. Monthly generator load test: Last completed 33 days before the date of the review by the hospital facility manager
d. Automatic standpipe flow test: Last completed 1 year and 2 months before the date of the review by the hospital facility manager

94. What are the ventilation requirements set by the American Society of Heating, Refrigerating, and Air-Conditioning Engineers (ASHRAE) for hospital airborne infection isolation rooms (AIIRs)?

a. They must be negatively pressurized, must exhaust 100% of their air supply, and must be provided with at least 12 air changes per hour (ACH) (2 of which must be fresh air).
b. They must be positively pressurized, may recirculate up to 20% of their air supply, and must be provided with at least 12 air changes per hour (ACH) (2 of which must be fresh air).
c. They must be negatively pressurized and must be provided with at least 20 air changes per hour (ACH) (4 of which must be fresh air).
d. They must be positively pressurized and must be provided with at least 20 air changes per hour (ACH) (4 of which must be fresh air).

95. A hospital facility manager has been tasked by senior leadership to benchmark the hospital's energy cost against an industry standard. Which of the following choices would NOT be a good benchmark?

a. Energy Use Intensity (EUI)
b. Energy Cost Intensity (ECI)
c. Building Energy Quotient (BEQ)
d. Power Usage Effectiveness (PUE)

96. How often should a master alarm panel for a hospital bulk oxygen supply system be tested, and what should be checked?

a. The master alarm control panel should be tested annually. The main tank low-level alarm, reserve tank in use alarm, and reserve tank low-level alarm should be checked.
b. The master alarm control panel should be tested quarterly. The main tank low temperature alarm, main tank high-temperature alarm, and reserve tank in use alarm should be checked.
c. The master alarm control panel should be tested monthly. The main tank low-level alarm, reserve tank in use alarm, and reserve tank low-level alarm should be checked.
d. The master alarm control panel should be tested every six months. The main tank low temperature alarm, main tank high-temperature alarm, and reserve tank in use alarm should be checked.

97. What unit measures sound intensity for the portion of the audio spectrum that human beings can hear?

a. Hertz
b. Phonon
c. dBA
d. dB

98. Which of the following statements regarding hyperbaric chambers is accurate?

a. Hyperbaric chambers increase interior air pressure to levels above atmospheric pressure. These chambers also increase oxygen levels above the normal atmospheric level.
b. Hyperbaric chambers decrease interior air pressure to levels below atmospheric pressure. These chambers also increase oxygen levels above the normal atmospheric level.
c. Hyperbaric chambers increase interior air pressure to levels above atmospheric pressure. These chambers also decrease nitrogen gas levels below the normal atmospheric level.
d. Hyperbaric chambers decrease interior air pressure to levels below atmospheric pressure. These chambers also increase nitrogen gas levels above the normal atmospheric level.

99. A common water management program control point for hospitals is the amount of residual disinfectant in the potable water supplied to the hospital by the local water utility company. Where should potable water be sampled from to best measure the effectiveness of this residual disinfectant in preventing hospital-acquired infections from waterborne pathogens?

a. It should be measured as close as possible to the point of entry to the facility.
b. It should be measured at the distal point of use.
c. It should be measured in patient showers.
d. It should be measured in cooling tower water.

100. How is the ability of a light source to faithfully reproduce colors measured?

a. The ability of a light source to faithfully reproduce colors is measured in lumens.
b. The ability of a light source to faithfully reproduce colors is measured by the color rendering index.
c. The ability of a light source to faithfully reproduce colors is measured by the chroma rendering index.
d. The ability of a light source to faithfully reproduce colors is measured by chroma.

101. Surveys of the physical environments of hospitals by accrediting organizations focus on requirements mandated by CMS K-Tags. Which of the following statements regarding CMS-K Tags is correct?

a. CMS K-Tag requirements come from the 2010 edition of the National Fire Alarm and Signaling Code (NFPA 72) and the 2010 edition of the Standard for the Inspection, Testing, and Maintenance of Water-Based Fire Protection Systems (NFPA 25). If a health care facility complies with these requirements, then its patients, staff, and visitors benefit from things like smoke detection systems, quick response sprinklers, initiation of fire alarms by sprinkler flow switches, and reliable transmission of fire alarms to emergency responders.
b. CMS K-Tag requirements come from the 2010 edition of the Standard for the Inspection, Testing, and Maintenance of Water-Based Fire Protection Systems (NFPA 25). If a health care facility complies with these requirements, then its patients, staff, and visitors benefit from things like quick response sprinklers, functional sprinkler valve tamper switches, and reliable initiation of fire alarms by sprinkler flow switches.
c. CMS K-Tag requirements come from the 2012 edition of the Health Care Facilities Code (NFPA 99). If a health care facility complies with these requirements, then its patients, staff, and visitors benefit from things like unobstructed exits, functional fire and smoke doors, airtight smoke compartments, effective fire drills, and properly constructed fire-resistant walls.
d. CMS K-Tag requirements come from the 2012 edition of the Life Safety Code (NFPA 101) and the Health Care Facilities Code (NFPA 99). If a health care facility complies with the requirements, then the patients, staff, and visitors benefit from things like unobstructed exits, functional fire doors, smoke-resistant smoke compartments, safe medical gas systems, and reliable electrical systems.

102. A fire door assembly serving a storage room has been inspected by maintenance staff during their annual rated door inspection and was found to be deficient because the door does not latch positively. Which of the following Interim Life Safety Measures (ILSMs) would best mitigate the risk posed by the deficient door assembly?

a. Increase fire drill frequency.
b. Remove combustibles from the storage room.
c. Educate staff concerning the hazard.
d. Add another fire extinguisher.

103. How can hospital facility managers ensure frontline maintenance technicians are included in a Plan, Do, Check, Act (PDCA) continuous improvement cycle for an organization's computerized maintenance management system (CMMS)?

a. Hospital facility managers can accomplish this by scheduling regular computerized maintenance management system (CMMS) training for all maintenance technicians.
b. Hospital facility managers can accomplish this during the annual performance evaluation of all maintenance technicians.
c. Hospital facility managers can accomplish this by establishing computerized maintenance management system (CMMS) benchmarks.
d. Hospital facility managers can accomplish this by including a task on every work order task list that affords the maintenance technician the opportunity to provide feedback concerning the computerized maintenance management system (CMMS).

104. How often should double-walled underground storage tanks be tested, and what kind of test should be done?

a. Hydrostatic testing should be performed monthly.
b. Vacuum testing should be performed quarterly.
c. Interstitial leak testing should be performed monthly.
d. Tank-wall conductance testing should be performed quarterly.

105. A health care facility manager has been tasked to review new construction plans for a behavioral health wing. During the review, the manager notes that the plans call for the patient sleeping rooms to occupy two smoke compartments on the second floor of the new wing. Each of these smoke compartments will have an area of 23,000 square feet. What should the manager advise to leadership concerning this proposed arrangement, and what NFPA document should be referenced?

a. The manager should advise leadership that the arrangement is compliant and reference Chapter 18 of the 2012 edition of NFPA 101.
b. The manager should advise leadership that the arrangement is not compliant and reference Chapter 19 of the 2012 edition of NFPA 101
c. The manager should advise leadership that the arrangement is compliant and reference Chapter 19 of the 2012 edition of NFPA 101.
d. The manager should advise leadership that the arrangement is not compliant and reference Chapter 18 of the 2012 edition of NFPA 101.

106. What amount of oxygen triggers the Department of Transportation (DOT) vehicle-placarding requirements for the on-site transport of oxygen?

a. 1,001 gallons
b. 501 pounds
c. 1,001 pounds
d. 501 gallons

107. A hospital facility manager has been tasked to design a portable fire extinguisher inspection, testing, and maintenance (ITM) program that meets the applicable requirements for type ABC, stored-pressure, dry-chemical, portable fire extinguishers. What are two applicable requirements, and where can the manager find them?

a. Fire extinguisher hoses are required to be replaced every five years. A fire extinguisher inspection is required every month. The manager should reference NFPA 25.
b. Internal inspection is required every six years. A fire extinguisher inspection is required every month. The manager should reference NFPA 10.
c. Fire extinguisher gauge replacement is required every five years. A detailed annual fire extinguisher inspection is required. The manager should reference NFPA 25.
d. Fire extinguisher hose replacement is required every five years. A fire extinguisher inspection is required every month. The manager should reference NFPA 10.

108. An electrical one-line diagram shows dashed lines through multiple areas of the building. What do they represent?

a. Relays
b. Hidden conductors
c. Transformer locations
d. Circuit breakers

109. Which of the following items could NOT be included as a line-item expense on a capital budget?

a. $10,000 for maintenance technician uniforms
b. $10,000 for structural engineering services
c. $10,000 for safety consulting services
d. $10,000 for an annual generator load test

110. A hospital electrical distribution system must have an ___________.

a. essential electrical system (EES) that includes an emergency power supply system (EPSS) with Life Safety and critical branches
b. emergency power supply system (EPSS) that includes an essential electrical system (EES) with life support and critical branches
c. essential electrical system (EES) that includes the life support and equipment branches of the emergency power supply system (EPSS)
d. emergency power supply system (EPSS) that includes the Life Safety and critical branches of the essential electrical system (EES)

Answer Key and Explanations for Test #1

1. A: Per the 2012 edition of the Health Care Facilities Code (NFPA 99), paragraph 15.13.3.10.3, there must be, at minimum, one annual operating room fire exit drill.

2. C: The National Fire Protection Association (NFPA) Standard 25 states that internal inspections of sprinkler pipes should take place every five years. As such, a system that received an internal inspection in 2025 would need another in 2030. NFPA 25 recommends weekly inspections of control valves and gauges for pre-action, deluge, and dry sprinkler systems and similar monthly inspections of wet pipe sprinkler systems. Water flow alarm devices, valve alarm devices, control valves, signal devices, hydraulic nameplates, and fire department connections require quarterly inspections. Pipework fittings, bracing, information signage, spare sprinklers, sprinkler heads, and backflow prevention assemblies should be inspected on an annual basis.

3. B: The thick, white deposits are built-up minerals from the water, often referred to as scaling. Water hardness refers to the presence of dissolved minerals in water, primarily calcium and magnesium. When the water is heated, it leaves the minerals behind and causes scaling that can impact the efficiency of the boiler over time. This makes the hardness of water the primary quality to address when scaling is a concern. Water with a balanced pH is less likely to cause scaling than water that is too acidic or too alkaline; however, this is due to the reaction between the water and minerals associated with water hardness. As such, it is more important to address the hardness of the water. Dissolved oxygen is the amount of oxygen present in water. It does not have a direct impact on scaling. Water conductivity is the water's ability to conduct an electrical current. The heat capacity of water refers to the energy required to raise the temperature of 1 gram of water by 1 degree Celsius. This has no bearing on scaling.

4. B:

Equation 1: $DS = PDR(PDC)(12)$

Demand savings per year (DS) [$/year] is equal to the product of monthly peak demand reduction (PDR) [kW] and monthly peak demand charges [$/kW/month] multiplied by 12 [months/year].

$$DS = 150(12)(12) = \$21{,}600 \text{ per year}$$

Equation 2: $ECS = ER(AES)$

Energy cost savings (ECS) [$/year] is equal to the product of energy rate (ER) [$/kW] and annual energy savings (AES) [kW/year].

$$ECS = 0.10(500{,}000) = \$50{,}000 \text{ per year}$$

Equation 3: $TAS = DS + ES$

Total annual savings (TAS) [$/year] is equal to the sum of the demand savings (DS) [$/year] and the energy savings (ES) [$/year].

$$TAS = 21{,}600 + 50{,}000 = \$71{,}600 \text{ per year}$$

Equation 4: $PB = PC/TAS$

Payback time [years]is equal to project cost (PC) [$] divided by total annual savings (TAS) [$/year]

$$PB = \frac{350{,}000}{71{,}600} = 4.89 \text{ years}$$

5. C: ASHRAE 209 is the best standard. Per the ASHRAE website: "To minimally comply with Standard 209-2018, building project teams must evaluate energy-efficiency options using modeling early in the design process (schematic design)."

6. C: The 2012 edition of NFPA 101 specifies that an ambulatory health care (AHC) occupancy requires a minimum width of 44 inches, and business occupancies require a minimum width of 36 inches.

7. B: A functional performance test runs the chiller under different loads, specifically to confirm capacity. Answer choice A is incorrect because an equipment schedule is a detailed list that typically doesn't contain any information about actual performance under load. Answer choices C and D are incorrect because they are reference books that do not measure anything.

8. D: To find the volume of 1 air change, first multiply the width, height, and length of the room. In this case, that would be $20\text{ft} \times 20\text{ft} \times 8\text{ft} = 3{,}200\text{ft}^3$. The required air changes per hour (ACH) per ASHRAE 170 is 12. That is equivalent to 12 air changes every 60 minutes, or 0.2 air changes every minute.

$$\left(0.2\frac{\text{air changes}}{\text{minute}}\right) \times (3{,}200 \text{ cubic feet}) = 640 \text{ cubic feet per minute (cfm)}$$

9. D: A dialysis machine malfunction can cause serious patient harm. The risk of serious patient harm falls under NFPA 99 risk category 1. Additionally, the test should check chlorine levels because chlorine is a disinfectant. Answer choices A and B are incorrect because total dissolved solids (TDS) tests do not measure residual disinfectant. Answer choice C is incorrect because the correct frequency for testing residual disinfectant is daily (before patients are dialyzed).

10. C: The 2024 International Building Code (IBC), Section 713 (Shaft Enclosures) states that shaft enclosures must have a fire-resistance rating of at least one hour when it is connecting less than four stories. Shaft enclosures connecting more than four stories must have a fire-resistance rating of at least two hours.

11. B: Economizers consist of a coil of metal tubes with a diameter of 1–2 inches that are placed in the outflow of the hot gases of combustion in the flue. Boiler feedwater is then circulated through this coil. The boiler water circulates from the boiler steam drum to the coil and then back to the steam drum. As the boiler water circulates through the coil, there is a heat transfer from the hot gases of combustion to the boiler water. This heat recovery results in as much as an 8% increase in boiler efficiency. Answer choice A is incorrect because economizers do not modulate combustion air. Answer choice C is incorrect because economizers do not employ plate and frame heat exchangers. Answer choice D is similarly incorrect because economizers do not use tube bundles.

12. C: Phasing plans are not legitimate grounds for any requests, as they are only plans. Errors and omissions in construction documents, unforeseen conditions, and owner-requested changes to floor plans are all legitimate reasons one may request a change order.

13. C: A failure of the emergency task lights cannot directly cause a generator failure. A malfunction of the day tank float switch, automatic transfer switch, or generator engine block heater can directly cause the emergency power supply system (EPSS) to fail to provide power during an emergency.

14. B: The annual cost recovery method calculates the equivalent uniform annual cost (EUAC) for each project alternative. It does this by assuming that each project alternative will be replaced until the end of the lifetime of the project alternative with the longest lifetime. Answer choice A is incorrect because even if the net present value (NPV) analysis is performed correctly, it may or may not generate the proper conclusion due to differences in project lifetimes. Answer choice C is similarly incorrect because it does not resolve the different lifetimes through an equivalency. As a result, it may also produce inaccurate conclusions. Answer choice D is incorrect because the internal rate of return (IRR) is the rate that is selected by a business organization to quantify the lowest acceptable rate of return on an organizational investment.

15. B: The correct answer is choice B because USC 42 §12188(b) gives this authority to the Department of Justice. Choice A is incorrect because the EEOC enforces employment-related ADA issues, not public space accessibility issues. Choice C is incorrect because OSHA enforces workplace safety regulations, not ADA regulations. Choice D is incorrect because the FGI is not an enforcement authority; it is a reference for facility design.

16. C: NFPA 99 establishes the Health Care Facilities Code that is used to categorize systems based on the risk of harm should the system fail. It divides the risks into four categories. Medical vacuum pumps assigned category 2 are considered moderate risk and have demonstrated the likelihood to cause minor injuries to patients, staff, and visitors should they fail. Equipment under Category 4 is not expected to have any impact on patient care. Category 3 equipment has been determined to likely cause discomfort to patients, but no injury. Category 1 is the highest risk and has the ability to cause major injury or death to patients and caregivers.

17. D: The criticality ranking of deficiencies facilitates prioritization; risk is proportional to criticality; and prioritization facilitates faster resolution of the most critical deficiencies (highest magnitude of risk) by enabling the resolution of these deficiencies before the resolution of less critical deficiencies. Answer choice A is incorrect because there is no relationship between the criticality ranking of deficiencies and the accuracy of root cause analyses. Answer choice B is incorrect because criticality ranking has no effect on funds available. Answer choice C is incorrect because criticality ranking does not reduce the total number of deficiencies.

18. D: If any project subtask is on the project's critical path and the duration is lengthened by a day, week, or month, then the completion date for the whole project will also be lengthened by a day, week, or month. Not surprisingly, there is more schedule completion risk associated with critical tasks than with noncritical tasks. Therefore, a delay in the completion of a critical task is never part of the best-case scenario for on-time completion. The best scenario is where the task in question is not on the critical path and, as such, cannot negatively affect on-time completion unless the delay exceeds the task's float (slack) time.

A phased-occupancy project schedule requires people to move in and out of occupied spaces while the project is ongoing. That means on-time project completion is dependent on people leaving existing spaces on time so demolition can get started on time and is also dependent on new spaces being ready to occupy on time so that the people vacating existing spaces for demolition have someplace to go. This adds complexity and risk to the project by introducing more points of possible schedule failure. Therefore, the best-case scenario for on-time completion is that the project does not employ a phased scheduling approach.

19. A: the total maintenance department budget is $1,000,000, and we know the maintenance department labor budget is 10% of the total budget, and 10% of $1,000,000 is $100,000; furthermore, we know the actual maintenance department labor budget is $125,000, which exceeds the budgeted amount by 25%.

$$\text{Maintenance department budgeted labor} = \text{BL}[\$]$$

Given that the maintenance department labor is 10% of the total BL, we have:

$$\text{BL}[\$] = 0.01(\text{total budget}) = \$100{,}000$$

$$\text{Budget variance} = \text{BV}[\%]$$

$$\text{Actual variance} = \text{actual labor expenditure} - \text{budgeted labor} = \$125{,}000 - \$100{,}000 = \$25{,}000$$

$$\text{BV}[\%] = \frac{\text{actual variance}}{\text{budgeted}} \times 100[\%] = \left\{\frac{(25{,}000[\$])}{100{,}000[\$]}\right\} \times 100[\%] = +25\%$$

20. B: The Center for Medicare & Medicaid Services (CMS) adopted the 2012 edition of the Life Safety Code (NFPA 101) on July 5, 2016. Chapter 2: Referenced Publications of this edition does indeed specify which edition of the other NFPA codes should be referenced.

21. B: The correct answer is B because seismic valves (earthquake gas shutoff valves) are the most effective method to mitigate this risk. Many localities in earthquake zones require their installation, and many earthquake insurance carriers require their installation before providing coverage.

22. D: Per paragraph 14.2.1 of the Standard for Installation of Stationary Pumps for Fire Protection (NFPA 20), all the fire pump major component manufacturers (or their factory-authorized representatives) are required to be present to witness the tests. Answer choices A and B are incorrect because the local fire department is not required to attend fire pump facility acceptance tests. Paragraph 14.2.2 of NFPA 20 simply requires that "all the authorities having jurisdiction shall be notified as to the time and place of the field acceptance test." Answer choice C is incorrect because the requirement is not found in the Standard for Inspection, Testing, and Maintenance of Water-Based Fire Protection Systems (NFPA 25).

23. B: Entry attendants may attempt rescue if they have been properly trained and equipped by their employer. Answer choices A, C, and D are all existing OSHA requirements that can be found in OSHA Standard 1910.146.

24. C: A power factor correction capacitor would allow the facility's electrical distribution system to supply the reactive current formerly supplied by the electrical utility. This may reduce electrical energy costs if the organization's electrical tariff penalizes low power factor. A power factor correction capacitor will reduce the current required for the total health care facility electrical load. This is important because heat losses are directly proportional to the square of the current, so power losses (and costs) increase exponentially as current increases linearly. Thus, a higher current is a nightmare for electrical utilities. It requires bigger conductors to maintain efficiency, and bigger conductors cost more money. That is why electrical utilities use a high-voltage (low current) transmission strategy. It permits the use of smaller conductors while maintaining efficiency, which reduces costs. While rebalancing loads would reduce neutral current in three-phase systems, this would not have any effect on the power factor. An inductor would lower the power factor, which would further increase the current required, making matters worse. Reducing the electrical load may or may not be effective (depending on which loads are removed), but it is typically not a practical solution. For more information, see the ASHE *Electrical Systems Handbook for Health Care Facilities* (Nash, 2013, page 32).

25. B: The provided American Society of Heating, Refrigerating, and Air Conditioning Engineers (ASHRAE) guidance is basic: if a facility tests, it must ensure the test lab is proficient in Legionella testing. Evidence of lab proficiency can be gathered through a certification from a government agency or an accreditation from a recognized accrediting organization. Answer choice A is incorrect because there is no 72-hour time limit for Legionella testing reports. Answer choice C is incorrect because there is nothing in the ASHRAE 188 Annex C guidance that mentions serogroup. Answer choice D is incorrect; while heterotrophic plate counts may be useful in identifying areas of biofilm that produce Legionella bacteria, ASHRAE 188 Annex C guidance makes no mention of these tests. See ASHRAE 188, Informative Annex C for more information.

26. B: Section 19.2.5.7.2.4 of the 2012 edition of the Life Safety Code (LSC) (NFPA 101) permits a travel distance of 100 feet from any point in the suite to an exit if the sleeping suite is protected by a sprinkler system.

27. A: NFPA 110 outlines performance requirements for emergency and standby power systems, such as generators. This standard outlines minimum preventative maintenance (PM) intervals for generators. NFPA 101 addresses the Life Safety Code, such as egress, emergency preparedness, and fire protection. NFPA 70 sets standards for safe electrical design, installation, and inspection. NFPA 37 focuses on the installation and location of stationary combustion engines and gas turbines. While this standard may guide the placement of a generator, it does not guide PM frequency.

28. C: An uninterruptible power system (UPS) is the only option that guarantees no power loss. A UPS is always supplying power and will continue to do so for a set amount of time after a utility power failure. A closed transition automatic transfer switch (ATS) needs a 100-millisecond overlap with utility power, so it would be unable to produce power if the utility power system has failed. A stored emergency power supply system (SEPSS) employs an ATS, so there will still be a brief power loss that accompanies unexpected switching. A ground fault circuit interrupter (GFCI) is used to shut down a circuit that has current leakage, not to eliminate switchover power loss.

29. A: Building Information Modeling (BIM) simulates spatial arrangements accurately enough to detect situations where an electrician might unknowingly run electrical conduit at the only possible location for HVAC ductwork. There are plumbers, electricians, fire protection specialists, and HVAC technicians who all utilize the above-ceiling domain to locate their work. It is very easy for one trade to encroach on another trade's installation location. The installation activities of all these trades must be coordinated to avoid installation location clashes. Answer choice B is incorrect because the pre-construction risk assessment (PCRA) does not consider the risk associated with trades coordination. It is more concerned with issues like noise and vibration. Answer choice C, the Critical Path Method (CPM), is incorrect because it is used for optimizing scheduling, not intertrade coordination. Answer choice D is incorrect because Interim Life Safety Measures (ILSM) are used to manage Life Safety risks generated by impaired fire protection systems and building features, not for intertrade coordination.

30. A: Emergency power is one of the most important requirements for continuity of care, and an inaccurate one-line diagram increases the risk of electrical failure that could cause injury or loss. Interim Life Safety Measures (ILSM) and infection control risk mitigation (ICRA) plans mitigate risks from Life Safety impairments and hospital-acquired infections, not power loss. Test and balance (TAB) is incorrect because it verifies that HVAC system performance meets design specifications concerning air pressurization of occupied spaces and cubic feet per minute of air supplied, returned, and exhausted, not power loss. Infrared (IR) imaging is helpful to predict failure, but it is not as critical as the accuracy of the one-line diagram, which is the basis for the design of the new electrical switchgear system.

31. C: Short cycling occurs when there are shortened refrigeration cycles due to improper heat transfers. While a clogged condensate drain line will leak into adjoining spaces and can harbor waterborne pathogens, it has no direct effect on the duration of the refrigeration cycle. By contrast, dirty air filters, a dirty evaporator coil, and low refrigerant levels can all directly cause short cycling.

32. C: A payment bond specifically guarantees subcontractors will be paid. Answer choice A is incorrect because a surety bond is an umbrella term for multiple bond types. A surety bond can be a payment bond or a performance bond, making it a less effective choice than a payment bond. Answer choice B is incorrect because a performance bond only ensures the completion of a project. It has nothing to do with subcontractor payments. Answer choice D is incorrect because a bid bond ensures the contractor will enter the contract if the contractor is awarded the project. It does not address subcontractor payments.

33. D: Per paragraph 8.2.2.4 of NFPA 25, the diesel fuel tank serving a fire pump diesel engine must be at least 2/3 full.

34. B: The National Fire Protection Association (NFPA) categorizes equipment as Condition 3 if it has missed the last two maintenance cycles, the last two maintenance cycles revealed issues, there are active or unaddressed monitoring notifications, or there are urgent actions identified through predictive techniques. Condition 3 equipment recommends that infrared thermography be performed every 6 months. Equipment that has been assessed as Condition 1 or 2 only requires infrared thermography every 12 months.

35. D: American Society of Heating, Refrigerating, and Air Conditioning Engineers (ASHRAE) standards are used to guide requirements for safe, efficient, and healthy indoor environments. ASHRAE 170 standards focus on ventilation in health care facilities, such as the air change rates in specific areas. The air change rate (the number of times the air volume of a space is replaced with fresh air in 1 hour) for a newly built airborne infection isolation room (AIIR) is 12 air changes per hour (ACH). AIIRs constructed prior to 2005 must have a rate of 6 ACH.

36. D: The Standard for the Inspection, Testing, and Maintenance of Water-Based Fire Protection Systems (NFPA 25) is correct because Chapter 14, Section 4 of the Standard for the Installation of Stationary Pumps for Fire Protection (NFPA 20) states, "Fire pumps shall be inspected, tested and maintained in accordance with NFPA 25." Answer choice A is incorrect because the Life Safety Code (NFPA 101) is more concerned with occupancy classification and the capacity of means of egress for evacuation than with the specifics of fire pump care and upkeep. Answer choice B is incorrect because NFPA 20, Section 4 of Chapter 14, specifically offloads upkeep to NFPA 25. Answer choice C is incorrect because the Standard for the Installation and Use of Stationary Combustion Engines (NFPA 37) applies to mitigating fire risk from stationary engines in general, not to the specifics of fire pump care and upkeep.

37. C: Answer choice C is correct because this falls under the 2012 edition of NFPA 101, Chapter 18 (New Health Care Occupancies), which applies to any health care occupancy built with plans dated on or after July 5, 2016. While Chapter 18 does permit the presence of certain wheeled medical equipment in corridors, it also requires at least five feet of unobstructed clear width when equipment is present. It is worth noting that this situation is compliant only if there is a hospital policy for relocating this equipment during a fire and staff members are trained and knowledgeable concerning their role in this policy.

38. B: There are four risk categories for hospital medical gas equipment established by the Health Care Facilities Code (NFPA 99). Category 1 is used to classify hospital medical gas equipment with the highest risk to patients and staff. A description of the four risk categories can be found in Chapter 4 of the Health Care Facilities Code (NFPA 99).

39. C: OSHA Title 29 CFR is where the information regarding the asbestos permissible exposure limit (PEL) is codified.

40. D: Answer choice D is correct because the facility condition index (FCI) provides data about the condition of capital assets and the relative priority for their repair or replacement. It is useful for scheduling asset replacement that avoids simultaneous expenditure of capital funds (budget spikes) for big-ticket items like roofs, chillers, and boilers.

41. B: Boilers are inspected and licensed annually by the state in which they operate. The license is contingent upon the correction of any deficiencies noted during the inspection of the boiler. Answer choice A is incorrect because boiler licensing is required every year, not every five years. Answer choice C is incorrect because there is no requirement for annual hydrostatic testing for boilers. Answer choice D is incorrect because not all jurisdictions require the presence of a licensed boiler operator.

42. D: The energy cost [C] [$] is the product of the hospital energy cost change per square foot [ECC] [$/ft^2] and the area of the hospital (A) [ft^2]. The energy cost change (ECC) is the product of the energy cost (EC) [$/ft^2] and the difference between the energy use intensity (EUI) [Btu/ft^2] before and after the chiller becomes operational.

Given: $EC = 0.012\left[\frac{\$}{\text{kBtu}}\right]; A = 1{,}500{,}000[\text{ft}^2]$

$$C[\$] = ECC\left[\frac{\$}{\text{ft}^2}\right] \times A[\text{ft}^2]$$

$$ECC\left[\frac{\$}{\text{ft}^2}\right] = EC\left[\frac{\$}{\text{kBtu}}\right] \times (EUI2 - EUI1)\left[\frac{\text{kBtu}}{\text{ft}^2}\right]$$

$$ECC\left[\frac{\$}{\text{ft}^2}\right] = 0.012\left[\frac{\$}{\text{kBtu}}\right] \times \left(95\left[\frac{\text{kBtu}}{\text{ft}^2}\right] - 80\left[\frac{\text{kBtu}}{\text{ft}^2}\right]\right) = 0.18\left[\frac{\$}{\text{ft}^2}\right]$$

$$C[\$] = ECC\left[\frac{\$}{\text{ft}^2}\right] \times A[\text{ft}^2] = 0.18\left[\frac{\$}{\text{ft}^2}\right] \times 1{,}500{,}000[\text{ft}^2] = \$270{,}000$$

43. B: The correct answer is choice B because section 7.2.1.9 of the 2012 edition of NFPA 101 requires electrically powered sliding glass doors to be "designed such that in the event of power failure the leaves open manually" in the direction of egress.

44. B: If a critical task has only two concurrently executed successor tasks, then one of those predecessor tasks must be on the critical path, as the critical path is continuous. Additionally, if one of these tasks has a longer duration than the other, then the longer-duration task is the one on the critical path. This is because, by definition, the critical path passes through the longest-duration task in a concurrent task set that contains it. In this case, task X's duration is tripled from 5 to 15 days. Task X will therefore have a greater duration (15 days) than task Y (10 days). Consequently, the critical path shifts to the longer-duration task X. Task Y can now be started anytime in the first five days without affecting the schedule's on-time completion, giving it five days of float time.

45. B: The correct answer is choice B because the new, more effective filters require more power from the air handling unit supply fan motor to maintain the required hospital airflows. If the air handling unit supply fan motor is not large enough to maintain the required airflows, airborne isolation rooms will be compromised, temperature control will not be effective in any occupied hospital space, and the required air changes per hour for surgical rooms will not be achieved. The other choices are not part of any mode of HVAC system failure related to installing more efficient filters.

46. B: To determine the compounded annual growth rate, the annual increase must be determined first by adding the Consumer Price Index – Urban (CPI-U) to the increase. In this case, that is 4+2, giving 6 as the annual rate. This is then plugged into the annual compound growth formula $[total\ growth\ factor = (1 + r)^n]$ where n is the number of years. In this case, the total growth factor would be: $(1 + 0.06)^3 = 1.191016$. Subtracting 1 and multiplying by 100 converts this to a percentage. $(1.191016 - 1) \times 100 = 19.1016$. This would round to 19.1%.

47. A: This facility is most likely located in a hurricane zone and must have windows that can withstand winds, heavy rain, and fast-moving debris. The American Society for Testing Materials (ASTM) sets international standards for a wide range of products and materials. ASTM E1996 specifies the performance of exterior windows, curtain walls, doors, and impact protective systems when subjected to windborne debris during a hurricane. As such, it is the most appropriate standard to apply to the windows of a facility built in a hurricane zone. ASTM E84 measures the surface burning characteristics of building materials. ASTM E1300 focuses on the load resistance of glass in buildings, specifically lateral loads like wind and snow. This standard is not applicable to hurricane winds. ASTM E8 sets test methods for the tension of metallic materials in all forms at room temperature.

48. C: As-built drawings provide the most relevant information of all the given choices. These as-built drawings will show in detail how fire and smoke barriers were actually constructed. The Life Safety drawings should be compared to the as-built drawings to ensure concurrence. For example, if the Life Safety drawings show a two-hour fire wall separating a health care occupancy from a business occupancy, then the as-built drawings should reflect that the construction of the wall followed the relevant design standard for a two-hour fire wall (such as two layers of 5/8 gypsum board). Answer choice A is incorrect because Life Safety drawings have nothing to do with suppression system hydraulic calculations. Answer choice B, while useful, is incorrect because health care facility evacuation diagrams are not as useful as as-built drawings. Answer choice D is incorrect because certificates of occupancy are not used in Life Safety drawings.

49. C: Per 14.2.4.5.4 and 14.3.1.4.5 of the 2012 edition of the Health Care Facilities Code (NFPA 99), the manager should check to make sure that fire drills are conducted annually and that fire drill documentation includes a measurement of the time required to evacuate a full complement of patients.

50. C: The coordination of mechanical, electrical, and plumbing (MEP) cannot proceed without details concerning clearances for maintenance access, utility requirements, and equipment dimensions. Subcontractor drawings provide the needed information and are the basis for MEP coordination. As an example, consider a hypothetical sterilizer installation and the possible implications of late coordination due to a lack of information provided by drawings. A sterilizer installation project requires, among other things, electrical power, a steam supply line, a condensate return line, and rigging. The rigger needs to know the dimensions of the sterilizer to plan its route so its movement to the install site is not impeded by door clearances. The rigger also needs to know the weight to ensure the elevator can handle the load. The electrician needs to know the power supply details provided on the drawings to provide the right overcurrent protection, conductor size, and voltage supply. Similarly, the steam fitter needs to know about the amount of steam required and how much condensate will be returned to size supply and return lines.

51. B: Per the Fair Labor Standards Act (FLSA), each week will need to be totaled separately. Any hours worked over 40 in either week should count as overtime.

52. D: The height requirement in each case is 36 inches above the finished floor (AFF); therefore, the front-approach counter is not compliant. This is referenced in sections 904.4.1 and 904.4.2 of the United States Department of Justice 2010 Americans with Disabilities Act (ADA).

53. C: Dashed conduit lines typically indicate a hidden conduit, or they can designate a conduit that is to be removed during project demolition. Since the manager is using as-built diagrams, there would likely be no representations of proposed demolition on this diagram. Therefore, answer choice C is correct. Answer choice A is incorrect because conduit bodies, unlike switches, are never mechanically linked. Answer choice B is incorrect because alternate feeds to automatic transfer switches are not represented by dashed lines. Answer choice D is incorrect because as-built diagrams do not include proposed demolition details.

54. B: The ventilation requirements for the design of airborne isolation patient sleeping rooms are provided in ASHRAE 170-2017. The ASHRAE 170 publication was rolled into the Facility Guidelines Institute (FGI) Guidelines publication in 2010.

55. B: For the four-hour generator load test that is required every 36 months, the test must be conducted for a continuous four hours, and the load must be at least 30% of the nameplate rating. The Joint Commission Standard EC.02.05.07 lists this requirement.

56. B: The Federal Emergency Management Agency (FEMA) Public Assistance Fact Sheet (2019 Revision) defines category E as public buildings and contents. Answer choice A is incorrect because category F is for public utilities, not hospitals. Answer choice C is incorrect because category B is for emergency protective measures, not mitigating damage to buildings and equipment. Answer choice C is incorrect because it covers roads and bridges.

57. D: Per OSHA Lockout/Tagout regulations, hospital staff must be trained in Lockout/Tagout procedures during orientation and annually thereafter.

58. B: The blended rate is the annual average total price rate in units of dollars per kilowatt hour (AATP [$/kWh]), and the cost avoidance (CA [$/year]) is the product of the AATP and the energy generated (EG).

EG = 1.2 GWh per year, or 1,200,000 kWh per year

$$\text{CA} = \text{AATP} \times \text{EG}$$

$$\frac{\$240{,}000}{\text{year}} = 0.20\left[\frac{\$}{\text{kWh}}\right] \times 1{,}200{,}000\left[\frac{\text{kWh}}{\text{year}}\right]$$

59. A: Medicare is an external factor, and the Strengths, Weaknesses, Opportunities, and Threats (SWOT) analysis framework examines Opportunities and Threats from external factors. The remaining answer choices are incorrect because they do not adhere to the SWOT analysis technique requirement to examine Opportunities and Threats in this context.

60. C: Dry burn is an event that represents the greatest possible risk a boiler poses: continued operation of a boiler burner when there is no liquid water present in the pressure vessel, resulting in a boiler pressure vessel explosion. There are five things that must fail in order for a dry burn to occur. There must be human error. There must be alarm failure. There must be a failure of the primary low water cutoff (LWC) and the secondary LWC. Finally, there must be a failure of the boiler makeup water system. The correct answer is choice C because a fuel pump failure would shut down the boiler burner. With the burner shut down, there would be no dry burn. Choices A, B, and D all add to the likelihood of a dry burn.

61. B: Answer choice B is correct per Annex A of the Standard for Emergency and Standby Power Systems (NFPA 110). Answer choices A and C are incorrect because the Health Care Facilities Code (NFPA 99) does not provide a sample form for documentation of monthly load tests. Answer choice D is incorrect; although NFPA 110 8.3.4.1 does establish permanent record requirements, these requirements do not address the specifics of a monthly load test, such as start time, end time, and restore auto mode.

62. D: Discounted payback periods consider the time value of money as an expense. Simple payback periods do not. Answer choice A is incorrect because both simple payback periods and discounted payback periods can include depreciation. Answer choice B is incorrect because discounted payback analyses do use the same interest rate. Answer choice C is incorrect because both simple payback periods and discounted payback periods can include taxes.

63. C: The quench vent exhausts liquid helium to atmospheric pressure at a safe location outside the building. It mitigates the asphyxiation risk to the building occupants due to oxygen displacement by helium gas. Answer choice A is incorrect because the risk mitigated is not MRI machine failure; it is asphyxiation. Answer choice B is incorrect because liquid nitrogen is not vented; liquid helium is vented. Answer choice D is incorrect about the gas vented and the risk mitigated.

64. A: Total dissolved solids (TDS) is the total amount of organic and inorganic material dissolved in a volume of water. Over time, these solids are deposited as scale on the waterside surfaces of the boiler. Minimizing TDS is the best way to prevent scale. Fewer solids dissolved in the boiler water means less scale formed on the waterside surfaces of the boiler.

65. A: The correct answer is A, H-1, per the FFA Advisory Circular 150/5390-2D. Option B is incorrect because category H-2 has an overall length between 15 meters and 24 meters. Option C is incorrect because category H-3 has an overall length between 24 meters and 35 meters. Option D is incorrect because there is no H-4 category.

66. A: According to AIA protocols, all minor construction defects on the punch list must be corrected, and the owner must have possession of all operation and maintenance (O&M) manuals for project equipment before final payment is requested. Hydrostatic testing is a disqualifier, as it has no bearing on final payment requests (it is a test for pressure vessel structural integrity). Answer choice C is incorrect because soil analysis and geotechnical survey are completed at the beginning of the project during planning. Answer choice D is incorrect because medical gas testing may or may not be applicable to a given project, and therefore, it cannot be a general requirement for final payment.

67. C: The manager in this scenario wants to compare the facility's Energy Use Intensity (EUI) to that of other facilities. To do so, the manager should access the EPA Energy Star Portfolio Manager. The Portfolio Manager provides percentile rankings and benchmark data regarding energy use for hospitals and acute care facilities. The CMS Hospital Quality Initiative Public Reports share hospital performance data related to patient care in a format that allows users to easily compare facilities. The Joint Commission Accreditation Database allows users to find organizations that have been accredited, certified, or verified by the Joint Commission. The American Hospital Association Annual Survey Database collects data on the demographics, operations, service lines, staffing, and other key metrics for thousands of hospitals and health care systems. This allows them to create comprehensive overviews of hospitals.

68. A: Estimates of profitability from methods of financial analysis that use the time value of money (TVM) are more accurate than those that do not. The net present value (NPV) analysis uses the TVM, so it will produce a more accurate result than methods of analysis that do not. Imagine the following scenario: you want to build a doghouse a year from today, and you know the price will be $100. You could put aside $100 today (at a price today of $100) or use the TVM to calculate the value of that money one year from today, which, if deposited in an interest-bearing account today, would yield the price needed ($100) one year from today. Given a positive interest rate, this price will always be less than $100, making it a more profitable choice. Answer choice B is incorrect because the annual cost method of analysis is used for alternatives with different lifetimes, and our alternatives have the same lifetime. Answer choice C is incorrect because the simple payback method does not consider the time value of money (TVM) in its analysis, so it will be less accurate. Answer choice D is incorrect because it only yields information about depreciation, so this analysis does not consider all relevant information.

69. A: Answer choice A is correct per the 2012 edition of the Health Care Facilities Code (NFPA 99), Chapter 3, Section 3, General Definitions. Answer choices B and D are incorrect because they reference external wiring, and the definition from NFPA 99 references internal wiring. Furthermore, answer choices C and D are incorrect because the definition of essential electrical system (EES) is found in NFPA 99, not the National Electrical Code (NEC) (NFPA 70).

70. A: Whether a project is completed on time and within the project budget are two of the most important ways to measure the effectiveness of construction project planning. Answer choice B is incorrect because the sustainability index is a fabrication, and energy benchmarks are statistics, not key performance indicators (KPIs). Answer choice C is incorrect because safety protocols and safety audit checklists are not KPIs; they are prescriptive tools for safety management. Answer choice D is incorrect; although the Energy Use Intensity (EUI) of the new space may or may not indicate effective planning, it is not as good a measure of this effectiveness as actual variance from budget and variance from actual completion date to scheduled completion date.

71. B: Answer choice B is correct because OSHA requires that a job hazard assessment be documented through a certification, not an identification (A and C). OSHA also requires documentation through a written document that self-identifies as an assessment certification. There are no requirements for the document to specifically list what was assessed or the method of assessment (D).

72. B: Discarded lamps and batteries should be classified as Universal Waste and may be accumulated for up to one year. The EPA Universal Waste Rule (40 CFR 273.15) governs the management of this waste. Answer choices A and D are incorrect because discarded batteries and lamps are not classified as Hazardous Waste. Answer choice C is not correct because Universal Waste may be collected and stored on-site for up to one year prior to transport to a recycling facility.

73. B: The punch list is used to track the resolution of minor construction defects during project closeout. Answer choice A is incorrect because a Certificate of Substantial Completion is not used to track the resolution of construction defects. Answer choice C is incorrect because a field observation report should be used during construction, not during project closeout. Answer choice D is incorrect because a warranty log is typically used after the project is completed, not to track the resolution of minor construction defects.

74. A: Answer choice A accurately describes a typical mode of failure for chilled water systems: cooling tower problems. In chiller refrigeration cycles, heat is transferred from occupied-space air to the chilled water loop by passing the air supplied to an occupied space through an air handling unit fan coil that is fed by the chilled water circulating loop. The chilled water leaves the coil at a higher temperature, and the air leaves the coil at a lower temperature. The warmer chilled water then continues to circulate to the evaporator, where it gives up its heat to high-pressure refrigerant, which is cooled by passing through an expansion device. The chilled water leaves the evaporator at a lower temperature, and the refrigerant leaves the heat exchanger at a warmer temperature. The warmer refrigerant then gives up its heat to the cooling tower condenser water in the condenser heat exchanger. The refrigerant leaves the condenser heat exchanger at a lower temperature, and the cooling tower condenser water leaves the exchanger at a warmer temperature. Finally, the heat is transferred from the warmed cooling tower water to the atmosphere by evaporative cooling in the cooling tower. The evaporative component of the system means there will be a constant need for water to maintain an adequate level in the cooling tower sump. That is why shutting off the cooling tower makeup water is such a showstopper. Answer choice B is incorrect because it describes the operation of a freeze stat. Freeze stat control sequences do not shut down chilled water. They protect coils from rupturing due to low outside air temperatures. Answer choice C is incorrect because static pressure low limit interlocks are not used to control cooling towers. Answer choice D is incorrect because outside air damper end switch interlocks are not used to control cooling towers.

75. C: The operative risk in this scenario is multiple patient deaths due to a fire alarm failure caused by service vendor negligence. Answer choice C transfers risk and incentivizes the vendor by making the vendor responsible if there are any malfunctions. The hospital wants each party to the contract to have some level of accountability. That way, the hospital's interests become the vendors' interests, too. The alternative (A) is incorrect because the service contractor would assume no risk and thus be less incentivized to reduce risk. Answer choice B is incorrect for the same reason as answer choice A. The vendor would assume no risk because the hospital indemnified the vendor from loss, and thus the vendor would be less incentivized to reduce risk. Choice D is incorrect because, unless the vendor indemnifies the hospital from loss, all risk is on the hospital, not the vendor.

76. D: Premium efficiency motors are most suited for static loads, and variable frequency drives (VFDs) are most suited for dynamic loads. Answer choice A is incorrect because the power factor is not a consideration in the question of a VFD vs. a premium efficiency motor. Power factor is largely irrelevant. Answer choice B is incorrect because ambient temperature is not relevant. Answer choice C is incorrect because VFDs are better for dynamic loads, not static loads.

77. D: An underground storage tank (UST) must be certified by an agency designated by the government of the state in which the UST resides. Most states use their Department of Environmental Protection. Answer choice A is incorrect because the Occupational Safety and Health Administration (OSHA) does not certify USTs. Answer choice B is incorrect because the Environmental Protection Agency (EPA) delegates this certification process to the states. The EPA does not certify USTs. Answer choice C is incorrect because the federal government leaves the designation of the agency that certifies USTs to the states.

78. B: Protective environment (PE) rooms should have a positive pressure differential of at least 0.01 inches of water column, and a manometer measures pressure differential. Answer choice A is incorrect because swing vane anemometers measure air velocity, not differential pressure. Answer choices C and D are incorrect because PE rooms should be positively pressurized, not negatively pressurized.

79. A: The best course of action is listed in answer choice A because adding capacitance to an electrical load with a power factor less than 1.0 increases the load power factor. This reduces the amount of current required to produce a unit of power, which reduces the per-unit cost of power over time (energy or kWh). Answer choice B is incorrect because it calls for installing the capacitor at the service entrance, not at the load. Answer choices C and D are incorrect because they call for an inductor to be installed, not a capacitor.

80. B: Developing a compliance strategy that complies with the most stringent of the codes in conflict increases safety for patients and resolves the conflict. Answer choice A is incorrect because CMS does not issue waivers for code inconsistencies. Answer choice C is incorrect because the Life Safety Code (LSC) does not take precedence over local codes. Answer choice D is incorrect; while it is technically true, it doesn't consider that not complying with the LSC jeopardizes Medicare funding for a hospital, which is typically over half of revenues.

81. B: The cracked sidewalk represents a hindrance to egress. K211 requires the exit discharge from a means of egress to be free of obstructions. K42 is a fabrication. K761 applies to doors, not sidewalks. K900 applies to NFPA 99, which does not address Life Safety issues. It focuses more on electrical and medical gas systems.

82. B: Waste gas scavenging is done in operating rooms to remove waste anesthetic gas (WAG) from the room's atmosphere to protect medical staff from being harmed by inhalation of WAG.

83. B: This was announced in a December 2013 Survey and Certification memorandum published by the Centers for Medicare & Medicaid Services (CMS). The memorandum says that health care organizations "may, through experience have identified more efficient and effective maintenance activities which do not reduce the safety of the equipment." The health care organization may deviate from recommendations through an Alternate Equipment Maintenance (AEM) program.

84. B: Lien waivers assure the lender that mechanics' liens will not be levied against the owner-borrower by subcontractors. Answer choice A is incorrect because the surety process guarantees an obligation will be met, not that project funds may be drawn without risk. Answer choice C is incorrect because subcontractor vetting is not a criterion for payment requests. Answer choice D is incorrect because a performance bond is produced by the surety process, and as detailed above, it is about guaranteeing that an obligation is met.

85. C: Answer choice C, International Performance Measurement and Verification Protocol (IPMVP), is correct per the US Department of Energy. Answer choices A and B are incorrect because they are communication protocols, not performance verification protocols. Answer choice D is incorrect because International Electrotechnical Commission (IEC) 62056 is a metering data protocol and not a performance verification protocol.

86. B: The correct answer is choice B per chapter 21 of NFPA 72, the Standard for Fire Alarms. The most frequent hospital elevator inspection, testing, and maintenance (ITM) interval is monthly testing of firefighters' emergency operation.

87. D: OSHA Standard 1910.147(c)(2) of Title 29 CFR codifies the requirement for an energy control program to control hazardous energy. Hazardous energy can take many forms: electricity, heat from steam in a boiler system, force due to air or water pressure, or even potential energy from gravity. If these hazardous energies are not dissipated or if their energy source is not locked out or tagged out, then employees are at risk. OSHA estimates 120 people die and 50,000 are injured annually from failure to apply Lockout/Tagout devices.

88. A: The value of chiller performance increased. Before the change, the chiller needed 0.65 kW of input power to produce 1 ton of cooling. After the change, the same ton of cooling required 0.9 kW of input power. Since the cost is directly proportional to electrical power input, and the electrical power input increases, the cost also increases. The percent of change is calculated by subtracting the initial value (0.65 [kW/ton]) from the final value (0.9 [kW/ton]) and dividing this difference by the initial value.

$$\text{Percent Change} = \frac{(0.9[\text{kWh}] - 0.65[\text{kWh}])}{0.65[\text{kWh}]} = \left(\frac{0.25[\text{kWh}]}{0.65[\text{kWh}]}\right) = 0.3846 \times 100 = 38.5\%$$

89. A: The acronym commonly used by staff to recall emergency actions for response to a fire is RACE: rescue, activate fire alarm, close doors, evacuate. Answer choice C is incorrect because it is the acronym for remembering how to operate a fire extinguisher, not the acronym for how to respond to a fire (that may or may involve an open flame that can be extinguished). Answer choices B and D are not commonly used acronyms.

90. B: The 2012 edition of the Life Safety Code (NFPA 101), Chapter 43 states that if an area of renovation is more than 50% of the area of a smoke compartment or greater than 4,500 square feet, then adjacent areas must be brought up to code.

91. A: The operative hazard in this case emanates from the presence of fungal spores, and air and surface sampling are the best ways to measure the level of fungal spores in the environment. Answer choices C and B are good things to do, but they do not assess the risk of the presence of mold. Answer choice D is incorrect because it only measures the concentration of particles in the air and does not specifically measure mold or spore concentration.

92. B: Per Appendix F to Part 112 of Subchapter D of Chapter I of Title 40 of the Code of Federal Regulations (CFR), the facility manager should include emergency response procedures and facility oil storage information. Answer choice A is incorrect because 29 CFR Part 1910 governs Occupational Safety and Health (OSHA) regulations. Answer choice C is incorrect because the Superfund Amendments and Reauthorization Act (SARA), Title III, is concerned with the cleanup of sites contaminated by hazardous chemicals. Answer choice D is incorrect because the Local Emergency Planning Committee (LEPC) does not govern the structure of response plans; the federal government does.

93. B: Dry system gauges should be inspected on a weekly basis in accordance with the 2011 edition of NFPA 25, page 13, paragraph 5.2.4.2. All the other records reflect compliance with their required schedules. Inspection, testing, and maintenance of fire and smoke dampers is required every six years in hospitals by NFPA 80. Standby generators should be load tested monthly per NFPA 110. CMS mandates that monthly load tests be performed no less than 20 days apart and no more than 40 days apart. NFPA 25 requires standpipe testing every five years.

94. A: Negative pressure, 100% exhaust, and 12 air changes per hour (2 of which must be fresh air) are all specified in Table 7-1 of the American Society of Heating, Refrigerating, and Air-Conditioning Engineers (ASHRAE) Standard 170. Answer choice B is incorrect because Table 7-1 specifically says that no recirculation is permitted and negative pressurization is required. Answer choice C is incorrect because ASHRAE 170 specifies 12 air changes per hour (2 of which must be fresh air), not 20 air changes per hour. Answer choice D is incorrect because it states that the room must be positively pressurized, but the ASHRAE 170 requirement is for negative pressurization.

95. D: Power Usage Effectiveness (PUE) is the ratio of total power used to the power used by the facility data center. It is a good benchmark of efficiency for facility data centers, but not for assessing the entire carbon footprint of a hospital. Answer choices A, B, and C are much better benchmarks because they consider the energy usage of the entire facility.

96. A: Answer choice A is correct per NFPA 99. Answer choices B and D are incorrect because there are no such temperature alarms provided for bulk oxygen systems. Answer choice C is incorrect because it says testing should be done monthly, not annually.

97. C: The correct answer is choice C because dBA is the abbreviation for decibels adjusted for human hearing.

98. A: Hyperbaric chambers increase oxygen levels and air pressure inside their chambers. Answer choice B is incorrect because it states that hyperbaric chambers decrease interior air pressure, but they actually increase interior air pressure. Answer choices C and D are incorrect because the hyperbaric chamber hazard is from an enriched oxygen atmosphere, not an enriched nitrogen atmosphere.

99. B: Residual disinfectant dissipates over time, so the worst-case scenario (in which the lowest level of disinfectant makes the water more likely to support waterborne pathogens) would be found at the most distant point of use. This makes the distal point of use the best place to measure the effectiveness of residual disinfectant. Answer choice A is incorrect because the best-case levels of residual disinfectant are found where the water first enters the facility. Answer choice C is effective in identifying risks to patients taking showers, but it is not a measure of the effectiveness of residual disinfectant in preventing domestic infections. Answer choice D is incorrect because cooling tower water is not potable.

100. B: The correct answer is choice B. The color rendering index (CRI) of a light source measures the ability of a light source to faithfully reproduce the colors that would be produced if the light source were the Sun. Humans' visual sensory bandwidth evolved to match the naturally available spectral content of the light source that dominates our environment: the Sun. Artificial lights do not have the same spectral content as the Sun. So, if one views a red car in sunlight, it appears red to the viewer. If one views that same car in a parking lot at night, and that parking lot is illuminated by a mercury vapor lamp, then it will appear brown, not red. This is because the light source (the mercury vapor lamp) is not emitting very much light in the red portion of the spectrum, so the human eye sees brown, not red.

101. D: Parts I and II of the Fire Safety Survey Report - 2012 Life Safety Code Healthcare (CMS Form 2786R) specifically reference the Life Safety Code (NFPA 101) and the Health Care Facilities

Code (NFPA 99). Answer choices A and B are incorrect because the National Fire Alarm and Signaling Code (NFPA 72) and the Standard for the Inspection, Testing, and Maintenance of Water-Based Fire Protection Systems (NFPA 25) are not directly enforced in CMS Form 2786R. Answer choice C is incorrect because it does not mention NFPA 101 as a source of K-Tag requirements.

102. B: The storage room's fire-resistant construction protects building occupants from what is inside the storage room, and removing the combustibles from the storage room effectively mitigates the fire hazard because there is no combustible material left in the room to support combustion. The other answer choices do not directly address the risk. Conducting more fire drills means people will be better prepared, but the risk remains. The same is true for staff education and adding a fire drill; these measures do not directly address the risk. If you could only do one thing, it would be to get rid of the fuel that would support a fire.

103. D: Hospital facility managers can accomplish this by including a task on every work order task list that affords the maintenance technician the opportunity to provide feedback concerning the computerized maintenance management system (CMMS). Answer choice A is incorrect because training does not necessarily imply feedback. Answer choice B is incorrect because an annual frequency would not produce timely feedback. Answer choice C is not a good choice because computerized maintenance management system (CMMS) benchmarks do not, in and of themselves, ensure maintenance technicians are included.

104. C: Answer choice C is correct per the Environmental Protection Agency (EPA); interstitial leak testing should be conducted monthly for double-walled underground storage tanks. Answer choice A is incorrect because hydrostatic testing is too involved to be done monthly, as it requires the underground storage tank to be emptied, filled with water, and then pressurized. Answer choice B is incorrect because there is no quarterly requirement for vacuum testing of underground storage tanks. Answer choice D is incorrect because conductance testing is performed on batteries.

105. D: NFPA 101 requires smoke compartments to be less than 22,500 square feet in area, and Chapter 18 of NFPA 101 applies to new construction. Answer choice A is incorrect because smoke compartments cannot be larger than 22,500 square feet. Answer choice B is incorrect because Chapter 19 of NFPA 101 only applies to existing health care occupancies, not to new construction. Answer choice C is incorrect because smoke compartments cannot be larger than 22,500 square feet.

106. C: This requirement can be found in 49 CFR Subpart F (172.504). Subpart F says that each container carrying any amount of hazardous material must be placarded. The only exception is for amounts less than 1001 pounds, not gallons.

107. B: The correct answer is B per NFPA 10. There are three requirements in NFPA 10 for type ABC, stored-pressure, dry-chemical, portable fire extinguishers: monthly inspection, a detailed annual inspection, and an internal inspection every six years. Answer choices A and C are incorrect because there is no five-year requirement for fire extinguisher hose replacement. Answer choice C is incorrect; while NFPA 25 *can* require gauge replacement every five years, NFPA 25 does not apply to portable fire extinguishers. NFPA 25 applies to inspection, testing, and maintenance (ITM) of water-based fire protection systems.

108. B: On a one-line diagram, dashed lines are used to indicate that the component is hidden or concealed within the walls or ceilings. They demonstrate the conduit path when it is not visible on the surface. Relays are indicated by a box labeled "R." Interlocking circles or coils are used to represent transformers. Circuit breakers are usually indicated by rectangles with a line through them to represent the interruption of power flow.

109. D: Capital expenses are major purchases like land, buildings, or machinery that are acquired to expand a business (like a hospital opening a new stand-alone emergency room). Capital expenses may also extend the useful life of an asset (like purchasing a replacement air-handling unit for a surgical suite in an ambulatory healthcare facility). Unlike operating costs, capital costs are not expended all at once; they are instead expended over the lifetime of the asset. The correct answer is choice D because the annual standby generator load bank test is part of the operations and maintenance (O&M) budget for inspection, testing, and maintenance (ITM). Choices B and C could be considered part of the capital budget if they are expended in support of a capital project. Choice A could be considered a capital expense if the uniforms are durable over several years.

110. A: An emergency power supply system (EPSS) is a subcomponent of an essential electrical system (EES) that provides backup power for the EES. Answer choices B and C are incorrect because there is no life support branch. This is typically a big point of confusion for people because they equate "Life Safety" with "life support," and power for life support medical equipment is backed up by the critical branch. Answer choice D is incorrect because an EES is not a subcomponent of an EPSS. It is important to understand the distinctions here because a health care facility manager's misunderstanding of the electrical distribution system terminology can cause patient harm.

CHFM Practice Test #2

1. Which of the following does a long-range capital investment strategy NOT provide?

a. Help for senior management related to understanding priorities
b. Information for employees about the facility's goals
c. Periodic review by an accountant and senior administrators
d. Help and direction for legal counsel and accountants

2. Which of the documents below is part of a submittal for a new MRI machine?

a. A load-bearing analysis that confirms floor capacity
b. Nuclear Regulatory Commission (NRC) design acceptance
c. Electrical safety testing of leakage current and ground resistance
d. Certificates of Calibration for test equipment

3. How does a service proposal with financials tied to the Consumer Price Index – Urban (CPI-U) protect owners?

a. By protecting owners from evergreen automatic renewal clauses in service contracts
b. By protecting owners from unreasonable price hikes in service contracts
c. By protecting owners from exclusions and omissions in service contracts
d. By protecting owners from litigation of service contract deliverables

4. What part of an AIA B101 agreement ensures construction documents are code-compliant?

a. Article 4: Liquidated Damages
b. Article 2: Architect's Responsibilities
c. Article 2: General Contractor's Responsibilities
d. Article 4: Owner's Responsibilities

5. Which of the following is NOT an alternative measure to save energy costs?

a. Replace mercury vapor lights with incandescent bulbs.
b. Draw light-colored drapes over glass areas at night.
c. Use infrared sensors to turn lights on.
d. Collect rainwater for watering plants.

6. What is a common method for managing risk arising from improper disposal of hospital radioactive waste?

a. The provision of dosimeters to affected employees
b. Lead shielding
c. Radiation portal monitoring
d. Use of a contractor for disposal of radioactive waste

7. How long do healthcare facility managers have to request reimbursement from the Federal Emergency Management Agency (FEMA) for expenses incurred during a presidentially declared emergency?

a. 60 days
b. 90 days
c. 45 days
d. 30 days

8. Which of the following construction documents lists the locations of electrical rough-ins for electricians?

a. National Electrical Code (NEC)
b. *IEEE White Book*
c. Equipment index
d. UL Listing

9. Hospital facility managers must ensure healthcare organizations have all the documentation necessary to prove compliance with the annual inspection of fire-rated doors requirement. What documents should hospital facility managers review to assess compliance with these requirements?

a. The manager should review life safety drawings, ILSM records, NFPA 80 training records, and the annual fire-rated door inspection report.
b. The manager should review life safety drawings, ILSM records, NFPA 101 training records, and the annual fire-rated door inspection report.
c. The manager should look for life safety drawings, ILSM records, NFPA 70 training records, and the annual fire-rated door inspection report.
d. The manager should look for life safety drawings, DOT records, NFPA 80 training records, and the annual fire-rated door inspection report.

10. The Centers for Disease Control and Prevention (CDC) lists four airborne infection-control precautions that impact HVAC design. Which of the following is NOT one of these four precautions?

a. Dilution
b. Particulate matter
c. Directed airflow
d. Building Pressurization

11. A hospital project management team is in the process of selecting a construction delivery strategy for an imminent project. If the health care organization wishes to maximize project cost certainty at the outset, then which of the following delivery methods should the team consider?

a. Design-Build (DB) and Construction Manager at Risk (CMAR)
b. Design-Bid-Build (DBB) and Construction Manager at Risk (CMAR)
c. Design-Bid-Build (DBB) and Design-Build (DB)
d. Design-Build (DB) only

12. What law requires wheelchair accessibility features in public buildings like hospitals?

a. SMDA
b. ADA
c. FMLA
d. CWA

13. Phase 1 of an energy management program involves:

a. Adjusting cooling and lighting
b. Setting up an energy database
c. Upgrading the facility's telephones
d. Changing operational practices

14. What points of inspection should be included on a hazard surveillance checklist for linen chutes in a five-story healthcare occupancy?

a. Is there a legible fire rating label on chute intake and discharge doors? Is the chute protected by a one-hour fire-rated door that latches positively on self-close?
b. Is there a legible fire rating label on the chute intake and discharge doors? Is the chute protected by a 90-minute fire-rated door that latches positively on self-close?
c. Is there a legible fire rating label on chute intake and discharge doors? Are the self-closing door and chute enclosed by a half-hour fire-rated barrier with no penetrations?
d. Is there a legible fire rating label on chute intake and discharge doors? Is the chute protected by a three-quarter-hour fire-rated door that latches positively on self-close?

15. A quad is:

a. A classification of biomedical equipment
b. A CAD architectural component
c. An electric demand controller
d. An extremely large amount of energy

16. Which of the following is NOT a component of the life cycle costing method?

a. The cost of the project divided by the cash flow
b. The amount of energy consumed during the project
c. Expected modifications and replacements
d. The initial investment in the project

17. When is a fixed foam fire extinguisher not required at a hospital helicopter landing area?

a. Fixed foam fire extinguishers are not required for helipads on occupied buildings that only serve H-1 type helicopters.
b. Fixed foam fire extinguishers are not required for helipads on unoccupied buildings that only serve H-1 type helicopters.
c. Fixed foam fire extinguishers are not required for helipads on unoccupied buildings that only serve H-2 type helicopters.
d. Fixed foam fire extinguishers are not required for helipads on occupied buildings that only serve H-2 type helicopters.

18. Which of the following is NOT an Interim Life Safety Measure (ILSM)?

a. Smoke barriers
b. Capped exhaust ducts
c. Fume hoods
d. Hand railings

19. Value engineering can be defined as:

a. A standard developed by the Department of Defense in the 1950s to deal with aging buildings
b. A tool for lowering costs by substituting equivalent materials that can do the same job
c. A slide show presentation to illustrate engineering proposals for a new facility
d. An assessment of electrical, plumbing, HVAC, structural, and fire safety systems

20. The Joint Commission (TJC) is:

a. A non-profit organization that provides information on rheumatic diseases
b. A new ADA regulation proposed by the Department of Health & Human Services
c. An organization that strives to improve patient safety
d. The agency which issues the final ruling in OSHA complaint cases

21. What is one intention of the Policy & Procedures (P & P) section of the Maintenance Manual?

a. To enable the CHFM to coordinate with emergency services
b. To aid HR departments when they are disciplining staff and preparing court cases
c. To prioritize measures that need to be taken during a power outage
d. To assist security in controlling access to equipment utility rooms

22. Which of the following factors is NOT commonly considered a risk to standby generator diesel fuel stored in tanks?

a. Intentional fuel contamination
b. Biological contamination
c. Water contamination
d. Short-term changes in temperature

23. One area that certified healthcare facility managers should concentrate their mold abatement efforts on is the:

a. Detoxification ward
b. Fuel oil storage tank
c. Nurse's station
d. Gerontology ward

24. The ability of a light source to faithfully reproduce colors is called the color rendering index (CRI). What is the recommended CRI for surgical lights?

a. 0–10
b. 90–100
c. 0–20
d. 85–100

25. Which of the following is NOT required by the ASME Safety Code for Elevators & Escalators?

a. Dumbwaiters should have signs indicating they are to be kept open for safety.
b. Freight elevators should have signs indicating the types of load they can carry.
c. Escalators should have signs telling parents to hold children's hands.
d. Passenger elevators should have signs indicating AIA compliance.

26. What is the key distinction between a submittal response of "approved as noted" and a submittal response of "revise and resubmit"?

a. "Revise and resubmit" and "approved as noted" both permit work to proceed, but "revise and submit" requires further documentation.
b. "Approved as noted" does not permit work to proceed, and "revise and submit" does permit work to proceed.
c. Neither permits work to proceed, but only "revise and resubmit" requires follow-up documentation by the subcontractor.
d. "Approved as noted" permits work to proceed, and "revise and submit" does not permit work to proceed.

27. Why was the Joint Commission's Statement of Conditions (SOC) developed?

a. To enable state or local authorities to enforce compliance with NFPA
b. To enable CHFMs to follow OSHA guidelines more easily
c. To help CHFMs create and maintain a fire-safe environment
d. To coordinate with the fire department for inspections

28. Calculate the life cycle cost (LCC) of an asset with an initial purchase cost of $2 million, a lifetime of 10 years, annual operations and maintenance costs of $16,000, salvage value ($1,000) equal to disposal cost ($1,000), no replacement cost, and an organizational minimum attractive rate of return (MARR) equal to 10%.

a. $2,098,320
b. $2,176,530
c. $2,068,440
d. $2,376,810

29. Which of the following would motivate a general contractor to bring a building project to completion at a lower cost?

a. A cost-plus fixed fee with upset figure contract
b. A cost-plus fixed fee contract
c. A cost-plus percentage contract
d. A guaranteed maximum price contract

30. What information best informs inpatient bed demand forecasting for health care facility master planning?

a. Centers for Medicare & Medicaid Services (CMS) forecasts
b. Demographics, such as market age cohort structure
c. Revenue projections
d. Geographic Information Systems (GIS)

31. Which of the following should be included in a service contract?

a. The year the company was established
b. The consequence of poor performance
c. A verification of energy consumption needs
d. Janitorial services for the entire facility

32. Which of the following is a characteristic of side arm water heating systems?

a. They are used with steam or hot water heating systems.
b. They are less efficient because of low recovery rates.
c. They are used to boost water temperatures for washing dishes.
d. They quickly provide large quantities of hot water.

33. A hospital is classified as a Small Quantity Generator (SQG). Under the EPA's Hazardous Waste Generator Improvements Rule, how long can the hospital go before re-notifying the EPA on their hazardous waste activities?

a. 1 year
b. 2 years
c. 4 years
d. 5 years

34. Which of the following devices is commonly used for managing hospital infection control risks from construction activity adjacent to occupied hospital space?

a. Photometer
b. Manometer
c. Balometer
d. Barometer

35. What portion of the audio frequency spectrum are humans sensitive to?

a. 5 nm–250 nm
b. 20 Hz–20,000 Hz
c. 10 Hz–1500 Hz
d. 20 nm–20,000 nm

36. Which of the parties entering a guaranteed-savings performance contract is responsible for measurement and verification of savings?

a. Commissioning Agent
b. Building owner
c. Energy service company
d. Electric utility company

37. If not repaired, broken coping can lead to:

a. Dust and pollen accumulation
b. Water damage inside the facility
c. A lapse in key monitoring
d. A clogged storm drain

38. The board of directors of a health care facility selects capital projects based on which of the following?

a. Changes in government regulation
b. Policies in the Operations Manual
c. Predictive maintenance procedures
d. An engineering assessment

39. Why are some CHFMs considering alternatives to traditional Intensive Care Units (ICUs)?

a. Because of the technological advances provided by bedside computing
b. Because patients in ICUs are more likely to get infections
c. Because ICU nurses are paid more than regular nurses
d. Because the Experts Committee published a document on ICU economics

40. How does a health care facility manager use the Energy Efficiency Ratio (EER) in financial analysis, and what are the units of this measure?

a. Health care facility managers use the Energy Efficiency Ratio (EER) to measure the operational cost efficiency of chillers. The unit of measure is the ratio of cooling output (Btu/hr) to electrical input (W), expressed as BTU/Wh.
b. Health care facility managers use the Energy Efficiency Ratio (EER) to measure the operational cost efficiency of buildings. The unit of measure is the ratio of the facility power usage (kBtu) and facility area (ft2).
c. Health care facility managers use the Energy Efficiency Ratio (EER) to measure the operational cost efficiency of boilers. The unit of measure is the ratio of boiler steam output (Btu/hr) and the facility area (ft2).
d. Health care facility managers use the Energy Efficiency Ratio (EER) to measure the operational cost efficiency of standby generators. The unit of measure is the ratio of power output (kW) per input kWh of electric energy, expressed as BTU/Wh.

41. Which of the following is NOT a responsibility of the safety committee?

a. Categorizing all accidents
b. Collecting input from employees
c. Filing claims for workers' compensation
d. Evaluating the results of an inspection

42. A hospital facility manager has been tasked by senior leadership to evaluate the hospital's energy cost with respect to an industry standard benchmark using the Energy Use Intensity (EUI) metric. Given a hospital industry standard benchmark EUI of 234 per kBtu per square foot (kBtu/ft^2) and the hospital EUI of 180 kBtu/ft^2, what should the manager report in the evaluation?

a. The manager should report that the hospital is performing well because the industry standard Energy Use Intensity (EUI) is 30% higher than the hospital's.
b. The manager should report that the hospital is performing poorly because the industry standard Energy Use Intensity (EUI) is 30% higher than the hospital's.
c. The manager should report that the hospital is performing well because the industry standard Energy Use Intensity (EUI) is 23% higher than the hospital's.
d. The manager should report that the hospital is performing poorly because the industry standard Energy Use Intensity (EUI) is 23% higher than the hospital's.

43. Which hospital Accrediting Organization compliance framework is associated with ISO 9001?

a. CARF
b. HFAP
c. DNV
d. TJC

44. When are electrically powered, automatically controlled sliding doors not required to have a "push to open" feature for egress during power failures?

a. This feature is not required for doors serving areas that are not continuously occupied.
b. This feature is not required for areas with a calculated occupant load of less than 50.
c. This feature is not required for doors serving areas that are 100 percent sprinklered.
d. This feature is not required for doors serving areas that are provided with smoke detection.

45. Scope creep occurs when the scope of a project grows, but the changes that caused the growth do not align with the project goals. It is an undesirable process. What construction document is the most effective in preventing conflict and scope creep?

a. Construction charter
b. Construction specifications
c. Request for information
d. Punch list

46. It is not uncommon for labor unions to pursue collective bargaining rights for hospital facilities teams seeking representation. These efforts to organize labor can take weeks or months to play out. The process culminates in a yes or no vote by the work unit members on whether to unionize. The outcome could be either a rejection of the effort to organize or the unionization of the work unit. To comply with the National Labor Relations Act (NLRA), members of management are prohibited from certain acts during this process. What acronym provides healthcare facility managers with a mnemonic device for recalling prohibited management actions during this process?

a. TIPS
b. ICRA
c. PASS
d. BOMA

47. Which of the following risks is associated with improperly maintained linen and trash chutes during a hospital fire?

a. Delayed fire alarm activation
b. Smoke inhalation
c. Building collapse from structural failure
d. Means of egress obstructed

48. When is an indefinite quantity contract most often used?

a. When the contractor uses a job book while bidding on work
b. When in-house staff and contractors are being used and flexibility is needed
c. When repair work on flooring, walls, and ceilings of a facility is being done
d. When a facility outsources its management

49. What standard governs hospital heliport fire safety?

a. NFPA 99
b. NFPA 418
c. NFPA 70
d. NFPA 101

50. What is the total project budget for a renovation that has $3.2 million in hard construction costs, soft costs estimated at 24% of hard costs, and a 10% contingency?

a. $5,374,700
b. $7,345,600
c. $4,364,800
d. $6,345,200

51. Calculate the annual straight-line depreciation (SLD) rate for an asset with a useful life of 10 years, a salvage value of $200,000, and an initial cost of $2,800,000.

a. $220,000
b. $240,000
c. $260,000
d. $280,000

52. When writing an Evaluation Performance Standard (EPS), the CHFM must:

a. Allow for delays caused by unanticipated changes.
b. Collect and preserve maintenance information.
c. Schedule operating and maintenance training.
d. Describe standards at an appropriate level.

53. The Director of Plant Operations in a hospital is working in a salaried position, but he has been working long hours due to a maintenance issue. He requests overtime pay for this extra work. Which federal law should the hospital facility manager consult to determine if the employee is eligible for overtime?

a. FLSA
b. OSHA
c. NLRA
d. FMLA

54. Interstitial spaces allow a health care facility to:

a. Consolidate office space in one area for improved efficiency.
b. Stay within the budget for a new building project.
c. Improve security by separating high-risk areas.
d. Upgrade HVAC systems without impacting patient areas.

55. What is a baseline energy audit?

a. An incentive rebate for a project that is energy efficient and results in reduced costs
b. A point against which future measurements can be compared to determine if energy consumption is reduced
c. A subsidy offered by the US Department of Energy (DOE) for certain energy efficiency projects
d. A plan to monitor and control the load cycle on a building HVAC system over a period of time

56. Which reference standard provides guidance for the installation of hospital lightning protection systems?

a. NFPA 780
b. UL 96
c. NFPA 70
d. NFPA 99

57. The NFPA 101: Life Safety Code is:

a. Related to public access to laboratories, drug cupboards, and morgues
b. A Standardized Emergency Management System (SEMS) designed to accommodate a triage area
c. Related to construction, protection, and occupancy features that minimize fire-related dangers
d. About establishing routines that follow OSHA's Bloodborne Pathogens Standard

58. Which of the following Americans with Disabilities Act (ADA) compliance options can reduce the cost of compliance?

a. Make some areas "Fully Accessible" to occupants with disabilities.
b. Make all areas "Fully Accessible" to occupants with disabilities.
c. Make all areas "ADA Adaptable" to occupants.
d. Make some areas "ADA Adaptable" to occupants with disabilities.

59. What organization maintains a system for tracking incidents of fire in the United States?

a. NFPA
b. NFIRS
c. FEMA
d. CPSC

60. A full-time safety officer helps the CHFM to do which of the following?

a. Direct an in-house fire team
b. Develop a fire brigade
c. Protect patients from radiation leaks
d. Maintain the error reporting system

61. When do allocated funds become committed funds?

a. When the check is written to pay for the order
b. When the purchase order is written out
c. When the money is negotiated for another purpose
d. When the funds are reflected in the budget report

62. Which of the following would be included in an operating budget?

a. Custodial functions
b. Compliance costs
c. Water consumption
d. Seasonal expenses

63. HVAC workers who handle refrigerants containing chlorofluorocarbon (CFC) are required to pass a certification exam administered by which agency?

a. ADA
b. OSHA
c. EPA
d. NFPA

64. Which of the following is an application of radio frequency identification (RFID)?

a. Recording peak energy requirements
b. Monitoring HVAC systems
c. Communicating with caregivers
d. Reducing treatment errors

65. What level of sound in the workplace triggers the requirement for a hearing conservation program?

a. 85 dBA
b. 85 dB
c. 90 dBA
d. 90 dB

66. What are the three ways heat may be transferred in steam plants employing fire-tube boilers?

a. Induction, convection, and emission
b. Conduction, convection, and emission
c. Induction, convection, and radiation
d. Conduction, convection, and radiation

67. What three event categories are included within the NFIRS Cause of Ignition field?

a. Deliberate act, mechanical failure, and act of nature
b. Act of nature, human error, and mechanical failure
c. Deliberate act, human error, and act of nature
d. Mechanical failure, human error, and deliberate act

68. How is a stairwell smoke control system used to control the spread of smoke during a fire?

a. Stairwells control the spread of smoke by exhausting more air from the stairwell than is supplied to the stairwell (negative pressurization).
b. Stairwells control the spread of smoke by having smoke detectors installed at the top of the stairwell.
c. Stairwells control the spread of smoke by providing more air to the stairwell than is exhausted from the stairwell (positive pressurization).
d. Stairwells control the spread of smoke by having smoke detectors installed at the lowest point in the stairwell.

69. What is the purpose of ordering a post-occupancy evaluation 6 to 18 months after a major project is completed?

a. To identify equipment that is not operating at optimum efficiency
b. To generate an Operational Space Program document
c. To solicit opinions from disabled people who frequent the new area
d. To show changes on as-built drawings modified from their original form

70. A health care facility manager has developed six energy-saving projects, four of which have an ROI of 18 months, and two of which have an ROI of four years. Given that the health care organization's ROI threshold for approval of energy-saving projects is three years, how should the manager proceed to maximize the amount of project work approved?

a. Request approval of the four projects with 18-month ROIs.
b. Consolidate all work into one project and recalculate the ROI.
c. Request a budget variance waiver from the organization's CFO and submit all six projects for approval.
d. Use EPA Business Credit Grants to finance the projects with a four-year payback.

71. Which of the following practices is used when selecting a bid for goods and services?

a. Outlining circumstances under which the contract can be terminated
b. Selecting from a group of vendors who feature only brand name items
c. Eliminating those vendors who score below a pre-set level
d. Showing the contract to the facility's legal counsel

72. What are four points of inspection that should be included in maintenance procedures for hospital lightning protection systems?

a. Air terminals, disconnects, bonding, and grounding electrodes
b. Air terminals, down conductors, bonding, and grounding electrodes
c. Air terminals, overcurrent device, bonding, and grounding electrodes
d. Air terminals, down conductors, overcurrent device, and disconnects

73. Which of the following is NOT a characteristic of biometrics?

a. Biometrics uses mathematical characterization.
b. It may require reverse pressure.
c. Biometrics is a field of biology.
d. It includes using retinal patterns.

74. As a contract administrator, the CHFM is responsible for which of the following?

a. Issuing an RFP (Request for Proposal)
b. Authorizing paperwork necessary for payment
c. Drawing up a demolition plan
d. Forming a selection committee

75. A healthcare facility fire safety program should include all but which of the following?

a. Monitoring employee behavior during a fire
b. NFPA Code 30
c. Identifying and removing or controlling hazards
d. Intruder alerts

76. A CMMS (Computer Maintenance Management System) contains which of the following?

a. Engineering assessments related to code compliance
b. Information about service contractors
c. Estimates of capital equipment expenses
d. Parts lists and diagrams from manuals

77. Suppose a hospital mechanical room contains a machine that generates noise with a loudness of 75 dB. Further suppose that a second machine that also generates 75 dB has been installed in that room. Are the requirements for a hearing conservation program or for a halving of exposure time triggered?

a. The requirement for a hearing conservation program is not triggered. The requirement for a halving of exposure time is not triggered.
b. The requirement for a hearing conservation program is triggered. The requirement for a halving of exposure time is not triggered.
c. The requirement for a hearing conservation program is not triggered. The requirement for a halving of exposure time is triggered.
d. The requirement for a hearing conservation program is triggered. The requirement for a halving of exposure time is triggered.

78. Suppose hospital patients are at risk due to the approach of heavy smoke from a distant wildfire. Further suppose the hospital facility manager has been tasked by senior leadership to monitor conditions and make recommendations accordingly. What parameter should the hospital facility manager most closely monitor?

a. Airborne particulates inside the hospital
b. Air exchanges per hour in occupied spaces
c. Carbon monoxide in occupied spaces
d. Outside air temperature

79. Suppose a hospital facility manager has been tasked with eliminating the presence of pharaoh ants in a hospital. Which of the following options is the least desirable?

a. Application of insecticide
b. Application of ant baits
c. Sealing the interior finish gaps and cracks
d. Increased frequency of inspections

80. What is the order of magnitude construction cost for an addition of 6 operating rooms, given the parametric rate is $825 per square foot, and each operating room will have an area of 400 square feet?

a. $990,000–$3,960,000
b. $1,980,000
c. $1,980,000–$3,960,000
d. $990,000

81. A CHFM would need an in-house fire brigade in which of the following situations?

a. To coordinate emergency management with the community (i.e. fire, police, and EMS)
b. To develop an alternate plan when evacuation routes are blocked
c. When based at an isolation facility for patients with communicable diseases
d. When items are contaminated with infectious clinical waste

82. A health care facility manager has been tasked by senior leadership to recommend the best construction delivery method for a small, free-standing emergency care facility. The manager's leadership team is inexperienced in construction and currently has its hands full with managing an IT project to implement an electronic health care record system. What delivery method should the manager recommend and why?

a. Design-Build (DB) because this delivery method is less complex and more simply executed
b. Construction Manager at Risk (CMAR) because this delivery method sets a guaranteed maximum price (GMP)
c. Design-Bid-Build (DBB) because this delivery method is the traditional form of delivery
d. Integrated Project Delivery (IPD) because it emphasizes stakeholder collaboration in the delivery process

83. Which of the following is NOT an organization that has developed a Model Building Code?

a. UBC
b. SBCCI
c. RBC
d. BOCA

84. What is the OSHA short-term exposure limit (STEL) for noise in the workplace?

a. The OSHA short-term exposure limit is 80 Hz.
b. The OSHA short-term exposure limit is 85 dB.
c. OSHA does not have a short-term exposure limit for sound intensity.
d. The OSHA short-term exposure limit for sound intensity is 30 seconds.

85. Predictive Maintenance (PdM) involves:

a. Monitoring equipment to identify developing problems
b. Controlling the maintenance department's budget
c. Ensuring the terms of a warranty are fulfilled
d. Using the Internet to disseminate medical information

86. Which of the following is NOT a duty of personnel who handle medical gases?

a. Changing the fittings on the gas cylinders
b. Learning to recognize color-coded gas labels
c. Inspecting fittings before connecting them
d. Storing medical gas cylinders apart from industrial gases

87. A health care facility manager is performing an economic analysis of the profitability of a project to replace existing halogen-lamped surgical task lights with LED-lamped surgical task lights. The manager's data collection reveals the project cost is $150,000; the annual savings from reduced energy costs will be $6,500; the life expectancy of the LED-lamped fixtures will be 10 years; and the discount rate is 8%. Given this data, what is the net present value (NPV) of the project, and how does this value inform the manager's decision to recommend (or not recommend) that the project be completed?

a. The net present value (NPV) of the project is -$106,384. This negative NPV means the execution of the project would result in a loss of value. Therefore, the manager should not recommend that this project be undertaken.
b. The net present value (NPV) of the project is $106,384. This positive NPV means the execution of the project would add value. Therefore, the manager should recommend that this project be undertaken.
c. The net present value (NPV) of the project is -$112,110. This negative NPV means the execution of the project would result in a loss of value. Therefore, the manager should not recommend that this project be undertaken.
d. The net present value (NPV) of the project is +$78,216. This positive NPV means the execution of the project would add value. Therefore, the manager should recommend that this project be undertaken.

88. A health care organization has solicited bids for a project to replace a failed emergency generator. The process has yielded three bids. All the bids are between 15% and 20% above the estimated and approved cost of construction. What course of action should the organization's health care facility manager recommend to the organization's senior leadership?

a. Accept the lowest bid.
b. Reject all bids, revise the contract, and rebid the project.
c. Renegotiate with the two lowest bidders.
d. Revise the scope of the project.

89. A lack of predesign planning during the design phase of a health care facility can result in which of the following?

a. A physical plant that is capable of carrying the workload
b. An increase in the risk of infection in the facility
c. A project that is not consistent with the facility's capital investment strategy
d. A decision to renovate the facility because of disruption

90. If a health care facility manager wishes to evaluate the technical qualifications of bidders for highly technical projects when bid prices are evaluated, then which procurement method is appropriate?

a. Best value procurement (BVP)
b. Value engineering (VE) procurement
c. Just-in-time (JIT) procurement
d. Selective tendering procurement

91. A condition assessment is a tool for determining which of the following?

a. The feasibility of a facility relocation
b. A price ceiling for alterations
c. How to properly allocate and spend funds
d. How to plan and schedule maintenance

92. The facility manager is responsible for all of the following duties related to fire safety EXCEPT:

a. Making sure the sprinkler system has been inspected and tested
b. Hiring a fire contractor
c. Knowing where specific monitoring panels are located
d. Keeping a detailed log of fire training

93. After evaluating bid submissions for a construction project, a health care facility manager finds that all bids significantly exceed the approved budget for construction. What course of action should the manager recommend to leadership?

a. Renegotiate with the lowest bidder.
b. Reject all bids.
c. Accept the lowest bid.
d. Cancel the project.

94. Which of the following is a characteristic of socially responsible design?

a. The design is based on information gathered from visits to other facilities.
b. The design complies with HIPAA (Health Insurance Portability and Accountability Act) privacy laws.
c. The design should not significantly increase capital costs on a per-bed basis.
d. The design should allow for acuity-adaptable patient rooms for the critically ill.

95. What is the unit of measure for sound that is used to quantify loudness in a workplace?

a. uH
b. dB
c. Hz
d. mW

96. What is an enthalpy wheel and where is it employed?

a. An enthalpy wheel is a heat exchange device employed by a steam boiler system.
b. An enthalpy wheel is a heat recovery device employed by an air-handling unit.
c. An enthalpy wheel is a heat recovery device employed by a steam boiler system.
d. An enthalpy wheel is a heat exchange device employed by an air-handling unit.

97. How does a CHFM calculate the average payback potential of a project?

a. By adding costs into a fund for basic expenditures and charging departments for overruns
b. By dividing the cost of the project by the annual net cash flow the project is expected to bring in
c. By calculating the sum of the after-tax savings from the project and the depreciation expense
d. By delegating work that exceeds the specified price to allow for a quick response to a need

98. What is an advantage of the chargeback cost control system?

a. It encourages cooperation between different departments.
b. It allows a healthcare facility to develop energy reduction goals.
c. It allows the facility manager to set rates as he or she wishes.
d. It encourages department managers to be more aware of costs.

99. What NFPA standard governs the requirements for smoke control systems in hospitals?

a. NFPA 92
b. NFPA 101
c. NFPA 99
d. NFPA 25

100. Direct digital controls are used to:

a. Test fire protection systems and sprinklers.
b. Generate blueprints of electronic systems and microprocessors.
c. Enhance temperature management in areas not used 24 hours a day.
d. Introduce outside air into a building to improve air quality.

101. How can activated carbon air filters best be used to mitigate the effects of wildfire smoke on hospital interior spaces?

a. Add activated carbon air filters to the pre-filters in air handling units.
b. Add activated carbon filters to outside air intakes.
c. Add activated carbon filters to final (HEPA) filters.
d. Add activated carbon air filters over HVAC air supply vents in rooms in occupied spaces.

102. What does *dry burn* mean in the context of boiler operations and maintenance?

a. A low-moisture combustion process to provide more energy per unit of fuel consumed
b. A repeated ignition failure of a boiler burner
c. A boiler burner continuing to fire when there is no water in the pressure vessel
d. A condition caused by the transfer of radiant heat from the boiler vessel to nearby exposed combustible surfaces

103. Many hospitals use electrically powered, automatically controlled sliding doors at main entrances. These door assemblies must have an emergency "push to open" feature that allows building occupants to manually operate the door in the egress direction so they can exit the building if the automatic door system loses electrical power. What is the maximum amount of required force that is permitted by the NFPA to manually set a leaf of an automatic door system in motion?

a. 5 lbf
b. 15 lbf
c. 25 lbf
d. 50 lbf

104. A hospital facility manager has been tasked by the health care organization's CFO to provide the blended rate the health care organization pays for electricity. Accordingly, the manager reviews an electric bill and finds the energy rate was $0.10 per kWh, the delivery rate was $0.07 per kWh, the monthly usage was 50,000 kWh, and the bill was $10,000. What blended rate should the manager provide the CFO?

a. $0.17/kW
b. $0.20/kW
c. $0.17/kWh
d. $0.20/kWh

105. Which of the following is LEAST likely to be included on a punch list for a substantially completed project?

a. Equipment planning for an expansion project
b. Plugged condensate drain in HVAC unit
c. Cracked fascia over waiting room entrance
d. Missing hand railing in geriatrics ward

106. ASHRAE (American Society of Heating, Refrigeration, and Air Conditioning Engineers) recommends that a minimum of 900 cubic feet of air per hour be distributed through a newer healthcare facility to avoid:

a. Malfunctioning microprocessors on the HVAC system
b. High humidity levels in the ICU
c. Shutdowns of the utility system
d. Sick building syndrome

107. Facility blueprints are reviewed to determine which of the following?

a. The effectiveness of maintenance
b. The location of blocked roof drains
c. Space for additional insulation
d. Access control to utility rooms

108. Which of the following choices is not a requirement for hospital heliport design?

a. Heliports must have two means of egress.
b. When fencing is used, two gates must be provided.
c. Heliports must be protected by a fixed foam fire extinguishing system.
d. Heliport helipads must have landing zone perimeter lights.

109. AutoCAD is a program commonly used to:

a. Show an object as if the viewer were looking down from above.
b. Indicate features such as doors using specific symbols.
c. Save time and money when producing engineering drawings.
d. Allow a fire marshal to test fire alarms and sprinklers.

110. If an interim Life Safety impairment mitigation plan for a project to demolish an existing dropped ceiling in a healthcare occupancy calls for re-use of the existing sprinkler fire suppression, then what would be the most important question to ask?

a. Do existing pendent heads need to be replaced with upright heads?
b. Does the existing fire pump have enough spare capacity?
c. Is the existing fire pump on emergency power?
d. Are there smoke detectors in the area?

Answer Key and Explanations for Test #2

1. C: The maintenance department budget is reviewed by an accountant and has nothing to do with long range planning. A capital investment strategy does help senior management as well as all employees understand the priorities and goals of the facility. It also helps accountants and legal staff to focus on an overall strategic plan.

2. A: A load-bearing analysis that confirms floor capacity is required because MRI machines are heavy (four or five tons), and this weight is concentrated in a small area. No MRI machine submittal is complete without confirmation by a structural engineer of floor capacity. Answer choice B is incorrect because the Nuclear Regulatory Commission (NRC) does not accept designs for MRI machines. Answer choice C is incorrect because it is a description of a generic electrical safety test for cord-connected appliances and not part of any MRI machine submittal. Answer choice D is incorrect because up-to-date certificates of calibration are quality indicators for test equipment maintenance, not part of any MRI machine submittal document.

3. B: The Consumer Price Index – Urban (CPI-U) is tied to the inflation rate. The underlying assumption is that price hikes in line with the CPI-U are reasonable. Answer choice A is incorrect because there is no relationship between the CPI-U and contract renewal clauses. Evergreen clauses in service proposals are usually removed at the request of the customer. The same is true for answer choices C and D. There is no relationship between these items and the CPI-U.

4. B: Answer choice B is correct because it is stipulated in paragraph 2.2.3 of the AIA B101 agreement.

5. A: When possible, mercury vapor lights should be replaced with fluorescent lamps, which cost less to use. Drawing light-colored drapery over windows at night will reflect heat back into rooms and save energy. When practical, using infrared sensors to control lighting can save energy. Collecting rainwater to water plants and shrubs reduces water usage and saves money.

6. C: The correct answer is choice C. Typically, radiation portal monitors (RPMs) are deployed by hospitals in the vicinity of the facility loading dock area adjacent to the trash compactor and other waste storage areas. Once deployed, this monitor must be operationally supported by routing all waste leaving the facility such that it passes through the monitor's field of detection so an alarm can be activated. Choice A is incorrect because dosimeters measure employee exposure to radiation. Dosimeters do not play a role in managing the risk from improper disposal of radioactive waste. Choice B is incorrect because lead shielding is not used to manage the risk from improper disposal of radioactive waste. Lead shielding is used in hospital "hot labs" to safely contain small amounts of radioactive substances with short half-lives as their isotopes decay, rendering the waste non-radioactive and harmless. Choice D is incorrect because the use of a contractor for disposal of all types of waste is a common (if not universal) practice. Using a contractor for radioactive waste disposal does nothing toward managing risk from improper disposal of radioactive waste.

7. D: The correct answer is choice D. Healthcare facility managers have 30 days to request reimbursement from the Federal Emergency Management Agency (FEMA) for expenses incurred during a presidentially declared emergency. More information can be found in "A Quick Guide: FEMA Reimbursement for Acute Care Hospitals" provided by the Yale New Haven Health Center for Disaster Response and Emergency Preparedness.

8. C: The equipment index is a room-by-room list of equipment that trades use to plan their work. If, for example, an electrician sees that a laboratory freezer will be in a certain room in the laboratory, then the electrician knows to provide power to that location. Answer choice A is incorrect because the National Electrical Code (NEC) is an NFPA Code (NFPA 70). It is not a construction document. Answer choice B is incorrect because the *IEEE White Book* is a high-level design reference for engineers and does not provide guidance to electricians on electrical rough-ins. It is not a construction document. Answer choice D is incorrect because a UL Listing indicates a device has met safety standards and does not address electrical rough-in work.

9. A: The correct answer is choice A because life safety drawings show all fire-rated door locations, NFPA 80 training records show maintenance staff competency in fire-rated door assessment, and ILSM records validate that the healthcare organization followed its policy for assessment of life safety impairments documented in the annual fire-rated door inspection report. The other choices are incorrect because they do not include the four items of documentation included in choice A (and only those four items).

10. B: The Centers for Disease Control and Prevention (CDC) list dilution of contaminants, the directing of contaminants toward exhaust registers, pressurization of individual rooms and spaces, and the pressurization of buildings as four precautions used in HVAC design. Particulate matter is not listed as one of these precautions.

11. A: In the Construction Manager at Risk (CMAR) delivery method, the construction manager gives the owner a guaranteed maximum price. The Design-Build (DB) delivery method also provides more cost certainty at the outset because it uses a single contract for project delivery. These two delivery methods should be considered by the team. Answer choices B and C are incorrect because the Design-Bid-Build (DBB) delivery method can generate change orders (after the contract is awarded) that significantly increase project costs. Answer choice D is incorrect because it excludes CMAR, which provides a guaranteed maximum price.

12. B: The correct answer is choice B, the Americans with Disabilities Act (ADA) of 1990. Choice A is incorrect because the Safe Medical Devices Act (SMDA) regulates medical devices. Choice C is incorrect because the Family and Medical Leave Act (FMLA) regulates human resources procedures for employee medical leaves of absence. Choice D is incorrect because the CWA refers to the Clean Water Act of 1972.

13. A: Phase 1 of an energy management system involves implementing energy conservation measures that will result in minimal disruption. These measures may include adjusting cooling temperatures and lighting levels. Setting up an energy database is done before implementing measures to manage and conserve energy. Upgrading a telephone system is an improvement but is not related to energy management. Changing operational practices is part of Phase 2 of an energy management program.

14. B: The correct answer is choice B because all the information given is in accordance with the 2012 edition of the Life Safety Code (LSC) NFPA 101. Choices B, C, and D are incorrect because they list the wrong fire ratings. Linen chutes by nature must penetrate the floors of healthcare occupancies. Additionally, the floors of five-story healthcare occupancies must have two-hour fire resistance ratings. Finally, protectives for openings in two-hour fire barriers (such as floors in healthcare occupancies) must be rated for 90 minutes per the LSC NFPA 101.

15. D: A quad is a very large amount of energy, equivalent to 172.4 million barrels of oil. Biomedical equipment includes imagers, defibrillators, and heart monitors. CAD (Computer Assisted Design) is used by architects and engineers to facilitate design. An electric demand controller allows electricity to be passed from one device to another.

16. A: Dividing the cost of a project by the net annual cash flow is done to calculate the payback period, the length of time it will take to recoup the capital investment for a project. Energy consumption is a component and is used to calculate the project's cost throughout its life. Expected modifications and the initial investment are also used to calculate the life cycle cost, as is the disposal of the project.

17. B: The correct answer is choice B per the requirements of Chapter 5 of the 2011 edition of NFPA 418. Fixed foam fire extinguishers are not required for helipads on unoccupied buildings that only serve H-1 type helicopters.

18. C: Fume hoods are used in isolation rooms to control or reduce the risk of pathogens. They are not an Interim Life Safety Measure. Choices A, B, and D are Interim Life Safety Measures. Smoke barriers are mitigation measures to protect the health and safety of patients and staff during construction. Capping exhaust hoods is also a mitigation measure. Hand railings contribute to the well-being of occupants.

19. B: Value engineering was developed by General Electric during WWII when not enough traditional materials could be found to complete the assembly of B24 bombers and other materials were substituted, resulting in lower costs. The Department of Defense developed EPS (Engineered Performance Standards) in the 1950s to help with efforts to maintain war-damaged, older buildings. Slide show programs are software designed to help individuals make presentations to an audience. An engineering assessment is used to identify problems in facility systems, such as HVAC.

20. C: The mission of TJC, formerly called the Joint Commission on Accreditation of Healthcare Organizations, is to improve patient safety and quality of care. A, an organization providing rheumatic disease information, is not logical. The Americans with Disabilities Act (ADA) is administered by the Department of Justice. OSHA, mentioned in choice D, issues its own rulings.

21. B: The P & P section of the Maintenance Manual clearly states policy so maintenance personnel can make decisions in accordance with laws and codes. HR can discipline staff if they fail to comply with the regulations outlined in the P & P section. CHFMs coordinate with emergency personnel by conducting regular drills to simulate different scenarios. A CHFM's top priority in the event of a utility failure is to inform caregivers about what to expect so that patients will not be endangered, but priorities are not established in the P & P section of the Maintenance Manual. Key monitoring helps security control access to equipment utility rooms.

22. D: The correct answer is choice D. Many hospital above-ground diesel fuel storage tanks are installed outside and therefore often experience short-term temperature changes with no risk to fuel quality. Choices A, B, and C are all recognized as posing risk to diesel fuel stored in tanks. Some bacteria and fungi can consume hydrocarbons in the fuel and degrade its quality. Water (from condensation inside the tank) is a common diesel fuel contaminant in storage tanks. Hospital diesel tank fill ports are kept locked to mitigate the risk of intentional fuel contamination.

23. D: The elderly are very sensitive to mold and can suffer more serious consequences if infected. Other groups that are highly sensitive to mold are infants, pregnant women, and those with respiratory problems. Choices A and C, a detoxification ward and a nurse's station, would in all probability not contain members of the highly sensitive groups listed above. Choice B, a fuel oil tank, would not be an environment in which mold would grow.

24. D: The correct answer is choice D per the International Electrotechnical Commission (IEC) Standard 60601-2-41. A CRI between 85 and 100 faithfully renders colors such that surgeons can make subtle distinctions in the color of blood and tissue necessary during surgery.

25. A: Dumbwaiters should have signs saying they are to be closed when not in use. Freight elevators should have signs indicating if they are for freight only or can carry passengers also. Escalators should have signs telling passengers to hold the rail and to hold children's hands. The AIA (American Institute of Architects) is a professional association for architects, and passenger elevators should have signs indicating AIA compliance.

26. D: A submittal response of "approved as noted" permits work to proceed, and a submittal response of "revise and submit" does not permit work to proceed.

27. C: The SOC is a document that was developed to help CHFMs create a fire-safe environment and demonstrate compliance with the Life Safety Code. NFPA is a non-profit agency that publishes codes and standards; it is not involved with enforcement. OSHA is concerned with protecting worker safety. Coordinating with the fire department for inspections is the responsibility of the facility manager and is not mandated in a document.

28. A: The life cycle cost (LCC) is the present value of all costs. The present value of all costs is the sum of the purchase cost ($2,000,000) plus the net present value (NPV) of the uniform annual series of operation and maintenance (O&M) expenses ($16,000 annually for 10 years at 10% interest). Salvage value is a positive gain ($1,000), and disposal cost is a negative cost ($1,000). Salvage and disposal are executed at the same time (end of life), so they cancel each other out and do not need to be considered further. Replacement cost is zero, so that term in the equation drops out.

The general formula for life cycle cost (LCC) is:

$$\text{LCC} = \text{purchase cost} + \text{net present value (NPV) of operation and maintenance (O\&M)} \\ + \text{NPV of salvage and disposal} + \text{NPV of replacement cost}$$

$$\text{Purchase cost} = \text{PC} = \$2{,}000{,}000$$

$$\text{NPVRC} = \text{NPV replacement cost}[\$] = 0[\$]$$

$$\text{NPVS\&D} = \text{NPV of salvage and disposal}[\$] = 0[\$]$$

$$\text{A}[\$] = \text{Operation and maintenance cost}[\$] = 16{,}000[\$]$$

$$\text{i} = \text{MARR} = \text{interest} = 10\% = 0.1$$

$$\text{n} = \text{lifetime[years]} = 10\text{[years]}$$

$$\text{Net present value of operation and maintenance} = \text{NPVO\&M}$$

$$\text{NPVO\&M} = \text{A}\left\{\frac{(((1+\text{i})^{\text{n}}) - 1)}{\text{i}(1+\text{i})^{\text{n}}}\right\}$$

$$\text{NPVO\&M} = \$16{,}000\left\{\frac{(((1+0.1)^{10}) - 1)}{0.1(1+0.1)^{10}}\right\} = \$98{,}320$$

$$\text{LCC} = \text{PC} + \text{NPVO\&M} + \text{NPVS\&D} + \text{NPVRC} = \$2{,}000{,}000 + \$98{,}320 + \$0 + 0\$ = \$2{,}098{,}320$$

29. D: A guaranteed maximum price contract fixes the maximum price for a project and would encourage a contractor to complete the job at a lower cost. A cost-plus fixed fee with upset figure contract sets a ceiling but allows the contractor to make a profit if costs are lower than the ceiling. A cost-plus fixed fee contract limits the ceiling and sets the profit margin. A cost-plus percentage contract allows a percentage for overhead and profit but does not motivate the contractor to cut costs.

30. B: The patient population is the key predictor. For example, if the local age cohort structure is top-heavy (lots of older patients, fewer younger patients), then it is likely you will need more inpatient beds to serve an older (sicker) population until the "bulge" in the cohort structure ages out. Answer choice A is incorrect because CMS does not forecast. Answer choice C is incorrect because revenue has no effect on patient health. Answer choice D is incorrect because geography does not directly influence demand for health care.

31. B: A service contract should clearly state the consequences of poor or non-performance by the contractor. The year the company was established would be included on a bidder qualification questionnaire. Verifying energy consumption is a duty of the chief engineer. Janitorial services are included in the maintenance and repair budget.

32. D: Side arm water heaters provide large quantities of hot water quickly and are moderately efficient. Heat exchange water heating systems are used with steam or hot water heating systems and are less efficient during months when heat is not required. Water heater storage tanks have a low rate of recovery and are useful for boosting water temperatures.

33. B: Under the EPA's Hazardous Waste Generator Improvements Rule, hospitals classified as a Small Quantity Generator (SQG) must re-notify the EPA regarding their hazardous waste activities every four years. SQGs are quantified as facilities that generate somewhere between 100 and 1,000 kg of hazardous waste per month.

34. B: The correct answer is choice B because manometers are commonly mounted on construction partitions to monitor air pressurization. Negative air pressurization in construction areas ensures no air from the construction area will enter patient-occupied spaces. It is well documented that patients exposed to airborne construction dust risk fungal respiratory infection from *Aspergillus*.

35. B: The correct answer is choice B; most humans are able to hear sounds in the frequency range between 20 and 20,000 Hz.

36. C: The energy service company (ESCO) is responsible for the measurement and verification (M&V) of savings. Answer choices A and D are incorrect because commissioning agents and electric utility companies typically do not enter guaranteed-savings performance contracts. Answer choice B is incorrect because the Department of Energy (DOE) regulations do not stipulate that the building owner is responsible; instead, they stipulate that the ESCO is responsible for annual M&V of savings.

37. B: Coping refers to the capping and sealing of a wall area on a roof. If not properly sealed, the roof will leak. Dust and pollen accumulation is controlled with air filters. Security oversees key monitoring. A clogged storm drain on a roof or in a parking lot will back up until cleared.

38. A: A change in governmental regulations is one of the bases for allocating funds for a capital project. Policies in the Operations Manual are the principles of the facility; they should be written and available for review by accreditation surveyors. Predictive maintenance involves monitoring equipment to identify faults before they develop into major problems. A detailed engineering assessment is used to identify non-compliance with codes as well as problems with building systems.

39. B: Patients in an ICU are prone to infection because of the high humidity, warmth, and low lighting levels found in ICUs. Bedside computing merely offers care givers improved technology to reduce medication mistakes and the amount of time needed to do paperwork. While some ICU nurses may earn more than regular nurses, that would not be a reason to look for alternatives to ICUs. An Experts Committee is concerned with making decisions that allow a construction or renovation project to progress on schedule.

40. A: Health care facility managers use the Energy Efficiency Ratio (EER) to measure the operational cost efficiency of chillers. The unit of measure is the ratio of cooling output (Btu/hr) to electrical input (W), expressed as BTU/Wh. Answer choices B, C, and D are incorrect because the Energy Efficiency Ratio (EER) is a measure of heat removal capacity, and buildings, boilers, and generators do not involve heat removal.

41. C: The CHFM, not the safety committee, is involved with filing claims for workers' compensation. Safety committee responsibilities do include investigating and categorizing accidents to see whether they were caused by system problems or employee behavior. Employee input is collected to help establish safety programs. Conducting safety inspections and evaluating the results is an important responsibility of the safety committee.

42. A: Energy Use Intensity (EUI) in general is directly proportional to energy cost. In this case, the benchmark EUI (234 [kBtu/ft^2]) is higher than the hospital EUI (180 [kBtu/ft^2]), so the hospital energy cost is lower than the hospital industry standard, which means the hospital is performing well. The magnitude of the cost difference (CD) can be calculated as a percentage by dividing the difference between benchmark EUI and hospital EUI by the hospital EUI, then multiplying the result by 100. The algebraic sign of the result of the calculation indicates performance. A positive sign indicates good performance, and a negative sign indicates poor performance.

$$\text{CD} = \left\{\left[\frac{(\text{benchmark EUI} - \text{hospital EUI})}{\text{hospital EUI}}\right](100)\right\} = \left[\frac{(234 - 180)}{180}\right](100) = 30\%$$

43. D: ISO 9001 is a standard that enables organizations to meet customer needs and comply with regulatory requirements in an environment of continuous improvement and efficiency. Accrediting Organizations (AOs) are bodies that validate that healthcare organizations receiving Medicare reimbursement from the US Treasury meet the Conditions of Participation (CoPs) for the Medicare program. This validation process is known as "deeming." Accrediting Organizations are authorized by Congress to perform audits (surveys) of healthcare organizations on behalf of the Centers for Medicare and Medicaid Services. The correct answer is choice D because the Det Norsk Veritas (DNV) website describes their accreditation standards as being "Aligned with NIAHO model and ISO 9001 principles."

44. B: The correct answer is choice B per Chapter 7 of the 2012 edition of the Life Safety Code (LSC) NFPA 101.Electrically-powered, automatically controlled sliding doors are not required to have a "push to open" feature for egress during power failures for areas with a calculated occupant load of less than 50.

45. A: A construction charter clearly delineates the project scope, purpose, budget, schedule, stakeholder responsibilities, and risks at the outset. This document provides a reference for the construction team to use as "true north." Answer choice B is incorrect because the specifications do not address the project scope. Answer choice C is incorrect because a request for information has no effect on project scope. It is simply an inquiry. Answer choice D neither reduces conflict nor prevents scope creep. It just lists minor construction defects that must be corrected.

46. A: The correct answer is choice A, TIPS, because employers are prohibited from *Threatening* employees, *Interrogating* employees, making *Promises* to employees, and *Spying* on employees. Choice B is incorrect because ICRA stands for Infection Control Risk Assessment. Choice C is incorrect because PASS is the mnemonic for portable fire extinguisher operation (Pull the pin, Aim the nozzle, Squeeze the handle, and Sweep the nozzle from side to side). BOMA is incorrect because it is the acronym for Building Owners and Managers Association.

47. B: The correct answer is choice B. The 1961 Hartford Hospital fire was caused by unextinguished cigarette ashes that were dumped down a trash chute. This ignited accumulated trash in the basement of the hospital at the chute terminus. The fire and smoke then spread through the chute to upper floors of the hospital, where 16 people died from fire and smoke. The other choices are incorrect because they are not related to Life Safety risk from linen and rubbish chutes.

48. C: An indefinite quantity contract allows the facility manager to order supplies and services for repair work to floors, ceilings, and wall areas. A job book contract is for work that exceeds a price already established. Mixing in-house personnel and outside contractors provides flexibility, and is known as body-shop contracting. A management contract is used when a healthcare facility is managed by a third party.

49. B: The correct answer is choice B because the title of NFPA 418 is the Standard for Heliports and Vertiports. Choice A is incorrect because NFPA 99 is the Healthcare Facilities Code. Choice C is incorrect because it is the National Electrical Code. Choice D is incorrect because NFPA 101 is the Life Safety Code.

50. C:

$$\text{Hard costs (HC)[\$]} = 3.2\text{ million[\$]}$$

$$\text{Soft costs (SC)[\$]} = 0.24(\text{HC[\$]}) = 768{,}000[\$]$$

$$\text{Contingency (CN)[\$]} = 0.1(\text{HC} + \text{SC})[\$] = 0.1(3{,}200{,}000[\$] + 768{,}000[\$]) = 396{,}800[\$]$$

$$\text{Total project budget (TPB)[\$]} = \text{HC} + \text{SC} + \text{CN}$$

$$\text{TPB} = \text{HC} + \text{SC} + \text{CN} = 3{,}200{,}000 + 768{,}000 + 396{,}800 = \$4,364,800$$

51. C: Straight-line depreciation (SLD) is the difference of initial cost (IC [$]) and salvage value (SV [$]) divided by the asset's useful life (UL [years]).

$$\text{SLD} = \frac{(\text{IC} - \text{SV})}{\text{UL}}$$

$$\frac{(2{,}800{,}000[\$] - 200{,}000[\$])}{10[\text{years}]} = 260{,}000\left[\frac{\$}{\text{year}}\right]$$

52. D: An EPS should be written so that a tradesperson will easily be able to understand it and complete the work that needs to be done. Allowing for unanticipated changes, absent workers, and weather means the CHFM must be flexible when drawing up a schedule. Collecting and preserving maintenance and repair information is accomplished with the aid of a computerized maintenance management system (CMMS). Before putting a new piece of equipment into use, training should be scheduled for all personnel who will be using it.

53. A: The correct answer is choice A. The Fair Labor Standards Act (FLSA) provides mandates on overtime pay and employee exemptions.

54. D: Interstitial spaces provide separate floors for electrical, mechanical, and HVAC services so maintenance and upgrades can be done without disturbing patient, treatment, and office areas. Interstitial spaces have nothing to do with office areas or improving security, and they add substantially to the cost of a new building project.

55. B: A base-line energy audit provides a point against which future measurements can be compared to determine if energy consumption has been reduced. Incentive rebates are offered by some utilities for projects such as installing more efficient heating systems. The US Department of Energy does subsidize renewable energy projects (solar, wind, etc.) in some states. Computers are used to control heating load cycles on building HVAC systems over time.

56. A: The correct answer is choice A because NFPA 780 is the standard for installation of lightning protection systems. Choice B is incorrect because UL 96 covers the manufacture of components of lightning protection systems, not their installation. Choice D is incorrect because NFPA 99 is the Healthcare Facilities Code.

57. C: The Life Safety Code is a document published by the National Fire Protection Association (NFPA) that sets standards to minimize danger from fire, heat, and toxic gases. Choice A refers to measures taken after an incident to prevent looting. SEMS is a standard for natural disaster preparedness, mitigation, response, and recovery. OSHA's Bloodborne Pathogens Standard is a routine that must be followed when dealing with hazardous waste.

58. D: The correct answer is choice D because the ADA permits some areas to be "ADA Adaptable." For example, for certain patient populations, not all patient exam rooms in a medical office require grab bars. A facility could certainly install these features in every room and be compliant, but it could also be compliant by installing just the support blocking during construction of exam room walls; this supports the potential future installation of a grab bar if patient demographics change. In this case, this option avoids the cost of materials and installation for the grab bars. Choice A is incorrect because making all areas fully accessible does not reduce costs but rather increases costs. Choice B is incorrect because not all areas are required to be ADA "Fully Accessible." For example, only one or two bathroom stalls in a public restroom may need to be "Fully Accessible" to be compliant. Making all bathroom stalls "Fully Accessible" is not needed for compliance, and it unnecessarily increases space requirements and labor and materials cost. Choice C is incorrect because making all areas "ADA Adaptable" is not compliant with the ADA requirements to have some areas be "Fully Accessible" and it unnecessarily increases cost by installing more "ADA Adaptable" features than are required by the ADA.

59. C: The correct answer is choice C because the National Fire Incident Reporting System (NFIRS) is a FEMA system. Choice B is incorrect because the NFIRS is a system, not an organization. Choice A is incorrect because the NFPA does not maintain a system for tracking incidents of fire. Choice D is incorrect because the Consumer Product Safety Commission (CPSC) does not maintain a system for tracking incidents of fire.

60. D: The safety officer helps the CHFM organize safety teams, assess risk, and maintain an error reporting system. Directing an in-house fire team is the responsibility of the chief engineer or the director of security. A fire brigade is a group of employees trained in accordance with OSHA standards to actually fight fires. Protecting patients from radiation leaks is an EMS duty.

61. B: A written purchase order that has been approved by the CHFM indicates that committed funds have been allocated. When the check is written, the funds are expended. When money is negotiated for another purpose, it is known as transferring funds through legal action. All three types of funds are reflected in a budget report.

62. D: Operating budgets include payroll, administrative expenses, supplies, taxes, insurance, and seasonal expenses such as lawn care. Custodial functions, such as trash removal, are included in a maintenance and repair budget. The cost of compliance with government regulations is in a management budget. Water consumption is part of the utilities budget.

63. C: CFCs are known to cause depletion of the ozone layer in the earth's atmosphere if released into the air, so the EPA (Environmental Protection Agency) administers the exam. A, ADA, or the Americans with Disabilities Act, is not an agency. B, OSHA, the Occupational Safety & Health Administration, oversees worker health and safety. D, NFPA, or National Fire Protection Association, has codes to reduce the risk of fire.

64. D: Patient care is one of the three applications of RFID, which can significantly reduce treatment errors and the administration of incorrect medications. Maintenance personnel monitor heating and cooling systems. A demand meter records the peak energy usage of a building. The CHFM bears the responsibility of communicating with caregivers in the event of a utility shut down.

65. A: The correct answer is choice A per OSHA (29 CFR 1910.25). Choices B and D are incorrect because decibels (dB) are not adjusted to match the portion of the audio frequency spectrum to which human beings are sensitive. The "A" in the abbreviation dBA stands for "adjusted," as in adjusted to conform to human audio frequency sensitivity. Choice D is incorrect because the number is wrong; the trigger number is 85, not 90.

66. D: The correct answer is choice D. Induction is incorrect because it involves magnetic fields rapidly changing their polarity to generate heat in ferromagnetic cookware. This technique is not part of steam plant operations. Emission is a general term with many usages. In general, it means "to send out." It is not used to define or describe heat transfer in a steam plant setting. Understanding heat transfer pathways is necessary for healthcare facility managers to oversee the effective and safe operation of boiler systems. An example of heat transfer by radiation is the Sun radiating heat. An example of heat transfer by conduction is the gradual warming of a cast iron skillet placed over a burner on a kitchen stove. An example of heat transfer by convection is provided by a lava lamp. Paraffin wax blobs in the bottom region undergo thermal expansion, which reduces their density. These less-dense blobs float to the top of the liquid chamber. The temperature at the top of the liquid container is cooler than at the bottom, so the paraffin blob becomes denser as it cools and sinks back to the warmer bottom region of the container.

67. A: The correct answer is choice A, per Section E of the FEMA Reference Guide. The other choices all include human error, which is not listed as a Cause of Ignition in the FEMA Reference Guide.

68. C: The correct answer is choice C because the positive pressurization of the stairwell space effectively prevents any smoke from entering the space. Additionally, as building occupants open stairwell doors to escape the fire, the air from the stairwell flows out from the stairwell, preventing any smoke from entering the stairwell and protecting the building occupants using the stairwell as an evacuation route from the lethal effects of smoke inhalation. Choices B and D are incorrect because smoke detectors do not control smoke. Smoke detectors simply initiate a fire alarm. Choice

A is incorrect because a negatively pressurized stairwell would suck smoke into the stairwell wherever a building occupant opened the stairwell door and would expose building occupants using the stairwell to evacuate to the lethal effects of smoke inhalation.

69. C: Soliciting opinions from staff and users of the facility, including disabled people, can measure how well the goals of a project were met. Determining this is a major purpose of a post-occupancy evaluation. Determining equipment efficiency to make sure there are no problems is the role of maintenance personnel. An Operational Space Program document provides the design architect with the information he or she needs to begin the schematic design for a project. As-built drawings are part of the design process and are derived from prints and other drawings.

70. B: The operative concept is to use the "low-hanging fruit" (energy-saving projects with quick payback) to leverage energy-saving projects with longer paybacks. The first step is to run the numbers again to see if consolidation of all six projects gets you over the ROI finish line. Answer choice A is incorrect because it does not maximize the amount of project work approved. Answer choices C and D are incorrect because EPA grants and budget variance waivers do not exist.

71. C: Before the highest-rated bid is selected, vendors are rated, and those who score below a pre-set level are disqualified. The contract is then awarded to the company judged to be the best. A and D both refer to service contract elements. Selecting from a group of vendors who feature only brand name items is a criterion for the lowest responsive bid.

72. B: The correct answer is choice B. Air terminals (lightning rods) receive the lightning discharge. Down conductors route the current from the lightning discharge to the grounding electrodes which harmlessly dissipate the charge into the earth. Bonding of metal ensures continuity of the safe current path from the tip of an air terminal to the earth ground. Choices A and D are incorrect because lightning protection systems do not employ disconnect devices. Choice C is incorrect because lightning protection systems do not employ overcurrent devices.

73. B: Respiratory therapy may require reverse pressure. Biometrics provides a positive identification of an individual through a template that is a mathematical characterization. It is a field of biology, and retinal patterns are one form of identification.

74. B: Authorizing paperwork for contractor payment is one duty of a contract administrator. An RFP outlines what will be done during a new building project. A demolition plan is completed to indicate which components of a facility will be removed during a renovation project. A selection committee is chosen during the first stage of a project to help choose a design firm.

75. B: NFPA Code 30 only establishes guidelines for the storage of flammable or combustible liquids. Choice A, monitoring employee behavior during a fire, is important so that patients and their confidential records are protected. C and D, identifying and removing or controlling hazards and intruder alerts, are crucial to fire prevention.

76. D: A CMMS contains information that has been scanned from various manuals, such as parts lists. An engineering assessment is done to help with maintenance issues. Information about service contractors can be obtained by talking to other health care facilities. Estimates of equipment expenses would be found in long range planning documents.

77. A: The correct answer is choice A because doubling a quantity that is used as an input to a logarithmic function does not double the output of that function. Instead, it increases the function output value (the new loudness in dB) by an amount equal to 10 times the logarithm of the factor of increase. In this case, the factor of increase is two because the amount of loudness present was doubled. Ten times the logarithm of two is approximately equal to three, so we can add 3 dB to 75 dB to yield the new noise level in the room of 78 dB. This value of 78 dB is less than the 85 dB that triggers the requirement for a hearing conservation program, so no hearing conservation program is required. Since the increase was less than 5 dB (only 3 dB), there is no halving of exposure time required either.

78. A: The correct answer is choice A. The risk posed by smoke from wildfires emanates from excessive levels of particulates in the air inside the hospital. Guidance from The Department of Health and Human Services (HHS) advises healthcare organizations to cease surgical procedures when indoor air particulate levels exceed 30 micrograms per cubic meter. The level of airborne particulates is therefore the best parameter of those listed.

79. A: The correct answer is choice A. Insecticide application is the least desirable because it is less effective and adds risk of chemical exposure for hospital patients, staff, and visitors. Choice B is a better option than choice A because ant baits are composed of an attractive food source that contains a slow-acting poison. Foraging ants return the ant bait to the ant colony where it is consumed by the queen. After the queen is killed, the ant colony dies. Choice C is a better option than choice A because if all gaps and cracks in the hospital interior can be sealed up, then the ants will have no way to get into the hospital. Choice D is a better option because no matter what plan is used to get rid of the ants, the facility manager will need to measure the effectiveness of the plan by frequently inspecting the area in question to determine whether the colony has been eliminated.

80. A: Order of magnitude cost is a range of costs from 50% of an estimate to 200% of that estimate. In this case, the estimate is obtained by multiplying the number of rooms by the square feet per room and then multiplying that square footage by the parametric rate. If you perform these multiplications, you get $1,980,000. The lower end of the range is 50% of that amount ($990,000), and the higher end of the range is 200% of that amount ($3,960,000).

81. C: An isolation facility not located close to EMS and fire personnel would be most likely to have an in-house fire brigade. Emergency management is coordinated through SEMS, the Standardized Emergency Management System. Facilities should always have an alternate evacuation route. Disposal of clinical waste is regulated by federal law.

82. A: The Design-Build (DB) delivery method is particularly suited for owners inexperienced with construction management. This is because DB uses a single contract and provides the owner with a single point of contact with the construction team (the general contractor). Answer choice B is incorrect because the Construction Manager at Risk (CMAR) delivery method was not designed for small projects. Answer choice C is incorrect because it is not a true statement. Design-Bid-Build (DBB) was not designed specifically for health care. Answer choice D is incorrect because it is a false statement. Integrated Project Delivery (IPD) works better with an experienced owner.

83. C: RBC stands for Royal Bank of Canada, which has not developed a Model Building Code. The Uniform Building Code (UBC), Southern Building Code Congress International (SBCCI), and Building Officials and Code Administrators (BOCA) are all organizations that have.

84. C: The correct answer is choice C because OSHA does not use the short-term exposure limit (STEL) for noise exposure. OSHA uses the STEL for exposure to chemicals. Instead of a STEL, OSHA uses a five-decibel exchange rate where exposure time is halved for every five-decibel increase in exposure.

85. A: Predictive Maintenance (PdM), also called condition-based maintenance, involves monitoring equipment to identify developing problems. The maintenance department budget is controlled through periodic reviews by the CHFM and an accountant. The facility manager is responsible for ensuring the terms of a warranty or guarantee are fulfilled. Using the Internet to improve the collection and dissemination of medical information is a strategy known as E-health.

86. A: Fittings on medical gas cylinders should never be changed. Maintenance personnel must memorize the color-coded gas labels to avoid connecting the wrong gas, which could result in injury or death. Fittings should be inspected before they are connected to make sure they are not worn, which could cause leakage. Industrial and medical gases should be stored in separate areas to avoid a mix-up.

87. A: The net present value (NPV) of this replacement project is the sum of the present value (PV) of the project cost ($150,000) and the PV of the uniform 10-year series of annual savings, where the amount of savings (A) is $6,500.

The present value (PV) of such a uniform series is calculated according to this formula:

$$\text{PV} = \text{A}\left[\frac{(((1+\text{i})^n) - 1)}{\text{i}((1+\text{i})^n)}\right]$$

The number of compounding periods (n) comes from the lifetime (10 years), and the value of i is the discount rate (8%). Plugging all these values into the formula and solving for present value (PV) yields a value of $43,616. That means the present value of a uniform series of annual savings of $6,500 discounted at 8% per year over a 10-year period is $43,616.

Savings are considered as positive cash flow, and costs are considered as negative cash flow, so when these values are summed to calculate the NPV, we have:

$$\text{NPV} = \$43{,}616 - \$150{,}000 = -\$106{,}384$$

For more information, see the latest edition of *Guide to Energy Management* by Capeheart, Turner, and Kennedy.

88. B: The bids were tight within a 5% band of variation. The astute health care facility manager will surmise that it is unlikely that all three bidders made mistakes in bid preparation that generated three very close bids. The manager will instead assume it is more likely that the bid package budget estimate is flawed, which means the design may be flawed. This means it is time to start over. Answer choice A risks completing a project with design flaws, so it is not a good choice. Answer choice C is not a good choice because the bidder left out of the renegotiation may litigate. Answer choice D is not the best choice because there is little wiggle room in the scope, given that this is an unscheduled emergency generator replacement.

89. C: A lack of predesign planning can result in a project that is not consistent with the organization's capital investment strategy and could cause an increase in operating costs. Carrying the facility's workload is a benchmark that surveyors use in accreditation. Infection Risk Control Assessment (ICRA) is employed to control the risk of infection in planning, design, construction, and maintenance. Facility disruption due to a lack of predesign planning would be related to building as opposed to renovating.

90. A: Best value procurement (BVP) looks at factors other than price, such as quality and expertise, when selecting vendors. Accordingly, this is the most appropriate procurement method because the best value for a highly technical hospital project may not be the lowest bid. For example, accepting a low bid from an inexperienced and less technically qualified bidder introduces additional project risk. Additional project risk reduces project value. Answer choice B is incorrect because value engineering (VE) is not used for procurement. Answer choice C is incorrect because Just-in-time (JIT) procurement is used to limit inventory, not to review the qualifications of bidders. Answer choice D is incorrect because selective tendering procurement just means bidders must be invited to bid.

91. C: A condition assessment is a tool for determining the effectiveness of maintenance and deciding how to properly allocate and spend funds. The feasibility of relocating a facility is determined by a relocation manager. Organizations set a ceiling for renovations and alterations to ensure an adequate percentage of funds are spent on repairs and maintenance. Detailed blueprints are used to help plan and schedule maintenance.

92. C: Knowing where specific monitoring panels are located is the responsibility of maintenance and operations personnel, not the facility manager. The CHFM should know the sprinkler system is fully operational, can hire a fire contractor or designate an in-house fire team, and must keep a permanent log of all fire training.

93. B: Until the bid package is re-examined and perhaps revised, it is best to reject all bids. See page 58 of *The Facility Manager's Guide to Health Care Project Management* (published by the American Society for Health Care Engineering) for more information. Answer choice A is incorrect because the cost overrun is significant, and every bidder exceeded the approved budget. This could mean there are problems with the bid package. Answer choice C is incorrect because there may be problems with the bid package, and accepting the low bid for a poorly designed bid package almost guarantees a contentious and difficult project execution. Answer choice D is not correct because project cancellation would not be in the financial best interest of the owner organization, and the effects of any existing functionally obsolescent building spaces will continue to hamper operations and negatively affect the organization's financial health.

94. A: Gathering information from visits to other facilities is one of the five characteristics of socially responsible design. HIPAA privacy laws mandate that telephones must be secure. Per-bed capital costs are taken into account when setting up a bedside computing system. Acuity-adaptable patient rooms are an alternative to ICUs.

95. B: The correct answer is choice B. Decibels (dB) are expressed using a logarithmic scale where the sound level in decibels (dB) is equal to 10 times the logarithm of the ratio of a sound's intensity to the sound intensity threshold of human hearing, where the sound intensity is measured in units of Watts/m^2 and zero (0) dB represents the threshold of human hearing. Choice A is incorrect because the microhenry (uH) is used to measure electrical inductance. Choice C is incorrect because the hertz (Hz) is used to quantify frequency. Choice D is incorrect because the milliwatt (mW) is used to measure power.

96. B: Enthalpy is the thermodynamic term for the total heat content of a system. (For this question, the system is the total heat content of a building.) Heat recovery devices capture heat that would otherwise be wasted. Heat exchange devices (such as shell-and-tube heat exchangers) transfer heat. Accordingly, the correct answer is choice B because some air-handling units (AHUs) employ slowly rotating heat transfer coils (enthalpy wheels) to *recover heat* from the AHU exhaust airstream and use that recovered heat to pre-condition the outside airstream as it enters the HVAC system. Enthalpy wheels can reduce the energy required to heat and cool a facility by over 25 percent.

97. B: The average payback potential is calculated by dividing the cost of the project by the annual net cash flow the project is expected to bring in. If the number of years calculated is equal to or less than a pre-determined time period, the project is acceptable. Adding costs into a fund for basic expenditures and charging departments for overruns refers to charge backs. Calculating the sum of the after-tax savings from the project and the depreciation expense is done to determine the actual payback potential. Delegating work that exceeds the specified price is done using a job order contract.

98. D: Chargebacks make managers more aware of costs and can lead to overall cost reductions for a facility. Chargebacks do not encourage cooperation between departments; they sometimes cause conflict. Allowing the facility manager to set rates is not an advantage of the chargeback cost control system.

99. A: The correct answer is choice A. NFPA 92 is the Standard for Smoke Control Systems.

100. C: Direct digital controls use microprocessors to save energy in numerous ways, including enhancing temperature management in areas not used all day. Fire protection systems are inspected by the fire marshal and the CHFM or a delegate, and alarms are tested regularly. Blueprints of mechanical and electrical systems are generated by CAD systems. Outside air is brought into a building to follow ASHRAE standards and avoid sick building syndrome.

101. B: The correct answer is choice B. This option protects the entire HVAC distribution system from contamination by filtering air at the contaminant point of entry to the system. The other options do not filter at the point of entry.

102. C: The correct answer is choice C. Dry burn is an event that represents the greatest possible risk a boiler poses: continued operation of a boiler burner when there is no liquid water present in the pressure vessel, resulting in a boiler pressure vessel explosion. There are five things that must fail in order for a dry burn to occur. There must be human error. There must be alarm failure. There must be a failure of the primary low water cutoff (LWC) and the secondary LWC. Finally, there must be a failure of the boiler makeup water system.

103. D: The correct answer is choice D per section 7.2 of the 2012 edition of the Life Safety Code (LSC) NFPA 101.

104. D: The blended rate is the total cost divided by the total usage.

$$\mathrm{BR} = \mathrm{TC/TU} = \left\{\frac{(10{,}000[\$])}{50{,}000[\mathrm{kWh}]}\right\} = 0.20\left[\frac{\$}{\mathrm{kWh}}\right]$$

Answer choices A and B are incorrect because they use [$/kW] instead of the correct units [$/kWh]. Answer choice C is incorrect because $0.17/kW is an incorrect value; the correct value is $0.20/kWh.

105. A: Equipment planning for an expansion project would not be included on a punch list of things that need to be done by a contractor. A plugged condensate drain would be included, as would a cracked fascia over a waiting room entrance. Essential items such as handrails that are missing would also be included.

106. D: Between 900 and 1200 cubic feet of outside air needs to be circulated each hour to avoid problems with indoor air quality in newer, more energy-efficient buildings. Quality problems can lead to sick building syndrome. Microprocessors are used to control elevator systems. High humidity levels in ICUs are a result of the low lighting levels found there. Utility shutdowns can occur because of emergency or scheduled maintenance.

107. C: Blueprints would be reviewed to determine whether there is sufficient space to add more insulation. The effectiveness of maintenance is determined by a condition assessment. Blocked roof drains would be identified by completing a visual inspection of the roof. Key cards or other types of identification would be used to control access to specific places in a facility.

108. C: The correct answer is choice C because NFPA 418 permits heliports on unoccupied structures that serve only H-1 helicopters (rotor diameters of less than 50 feet) to have two portable foam extinguishers instead of a fixed foam fire extinguishing system. Choices A, B, and D are required by NFPA 418 for all heliports regardless of the type of aircraft served.

109. C: AutoCAD (Computer Aided Design) uses special software to speed up the process of creating engineering and architectural plans, which saves time and money. A plan view is a blueprint that shows objects as if the viewer were looking down from above. Building blueprints use specific symbols to indicate features such as windows, doors, and electrical outlets. A fire marshal, accompanied by the CHFM or a delegate, regularly inspects fire alarms and sprinklers, but does not use any software programs to do so.

110. A: The correct answer is choice A because pendent heads are not designed to protect areas without dropped ceilings. The removal of the ceiling membrane significantly increases the volume of the room. That increase in volume requires more heat to be added to the space to activate the sprinklers. This delays their timely activation and increases the risk of fire spreading uncontrollably. Choice B is incorrect because this scenario involves an existing space, so no additional fire pump capacity will be required. Choice C is incorrect because all fire pumps are required to be on an emergency power circuit. Choice D is incorrect because smoke detectors are not part of a fire suppression system.

How to Overcome Test Anxiety

Just the thought of taking a test is enough to make most people a little nervous. A test is an important event that can have a long-term impact on your future, so it's important to take it seriously and it's natural to feel anxious about performing well. But just because anxiety is normal, that doesn't mean that it's helpful in test taking, or that you should simply accept it as part of your life. Anxiety can have a variety of effects. These effects can be mild, like making you feel slightly nervous, or severe, like blocking your ability to focus or remember even a simple detail.

If you experience test anxiety—whether severe or mild—it's important to know how to beat it. To discover this, first you need to understand what causes test anxiety.

Causes of Test Anxiety

While we often think of anxiety as an uncontrollable emotional state, it can actually be caused by simple, practical things. One of the most common causes of test anxiety is that a person does not feel adequately prepared for their test. This feeling can be the result of many different issues such as poor study habits or lack of organization, but the most common culprit is time management. Starting to study too late, failing to organize your study time to cover all of the material, or being distracted while you study will mean that you're not well prepared for the test. This may lead to cramming the night before, which will cause you to be physically and mentally exhausted for the test. Poor time management also contributes to feelings of stress, fear, and hopelessness as you realize you are not well prepared but don't know what to do about it.

Other times, test anxiety is not related to your preparation for the test but comes from unresolved fear. This may be a past failure on a test, or poor performance on tests in general. It may come from comparing yourself to others who seem to be performing better or from the stress of living up to expectations. Anxiety may be driven by fears of the future—how failure on this test would affect your educational and career goals. These fears are often completely irrational, but they can still negatively impact your test performance.

Elements of Test Anxiety

As mentioned earlier, test anxiety is considered to be an emotional state, but it has physical and mental components as well. Sometimes you may not even realize that you are suffering from test anxiety until you notice the physical symptoms. These can include trembling hands, rapid heartbeat, sweating, nausea, and tense muscles. Extreme anxiety may lead to fainting or vomiting. Obviously, any of these symptoms can have a negative impact on testing. It is important to recognize them as soon as they begin to occur so that you can address the problem before it damages your performance.

The mental components of test anxiety include trouble focusing and inability to remember learned information. During a test, your mind is on high alert, which can help you recall information and stay focused for an extended period of time. However, anxiety interferes with your mind's natural processes, causing you to blank out, even on the questions you know well. The strain of testing during anxiety makes it difficult to stay focused, especially on a test that may take several hours. Extreme anxiety can take a huge mental toll, making it difficult not only to recall test information but even to understand the test questions or pull your thoughts together.

Effects of Test Anxiety

Test anxiety is like a disease—if left untreated, it will get progressively worse. Anxiety leads to poor performance, and this reinforces the feelings of fear and failure, which in turn lead to poor performances on subsequent tests. It can grow from a mild nervousness to a crippling condition. If allowed to progress, test anxiety can have a big impact on your schooling, and consequently on your future.

Test anxiety can spread to other parts of your life. Anxiety on tests can become anxiety in any stressful situation, and blanking on a test can turn into panicking in a job situation. But fortunately, you don't have to let anxiety rule your testing and determine your grades. There are a number of relatively simple steps you can take to move past anxiety and function normally on a test and in the rest of life.

Physical Steps for Beating Test Anxiety

While test anxiety is a serious problem, the good news is that it can be overcome. It doesn't have to control your ability to think and remember information. While it may take time, you can begin taking steps today to beat anxiety.

Just as your first hint that you may be struggling with anxiety comes from the physical symptoms, the first step to treating it is also physical. Rest is crucial for having a clear, strong mind. If you are tired, it is much easier to give in to anxiety. But if you establish good sleep habits, your body and mind will be ready to perform optimally, without the strain of exhaustion. Additionally, sleeping well helps you to retain information better, so you're more likely to recall the answers when you see the test questions.

Getting good sleep means more than going to bed on time. It's important to allow your brain time to relax. Take study breaks from time to time so it doesn't get overworked, and don't study right before bed. Take time to rest your mind before trying to rest your body, or you may find it difficult to fall asleep.

Along with sleep, other aspects of physical health are important in preparing for a test. Good nutrition is vital for good brain function. Sugary foods and drinks may give a burst of energy but this burst is followed by a crash, both physically and emotionally. Instead, fuel your body with protein and vitamin-rich foods.

Also, drink plenty of water. Dehydration can lead to headaches and exhaustion, especially if your brain is already under stress from the rigors of the test. Particularly if your test is a long one, drink water during the breaks. And if possible, take an energy-boosting snack to eat between sections.

Along with sleep and diet, a third important part of physical health is exercise. Maintaining a steady workout schedule is helpful, but even taking 5-minute study breaks to walk can help get your blood pumping faster and clear your head. Exercise also releases endorphins, which contribute to a positive feeling and can help combat test anxiety.

When you nurture your physical health, you are also contributing to your mental health. If your body is healthy, your mind is much more likely to be healthy as well. So take time to rest, nourish your body with healthy food and water, and get moving as much as possible. Taking these physical steps will make you stronger and more able to take the mental steps necessary to overcome test anxiety.

Mental Steps for Beating Test Anxiety

Working on the mental side of test anxiety can be more challenging, but as with the physical side, there are clear steps you can take to overcome it. As mentioned earlier, test anxiety often stems from lack of preparation, so the obvious solution is to prepare for the test. Effective studying may be the most important weapon you have for beating test anxiety, but you can and should employ several other mental tools to combat fear.

First, boost your confidence by reminding yourself of past success—tests or projects that you aced. If you're putting as much effort into preparing for this test as you did for those, there's no reason you should expect to fail here. Work hard to prepare; then trust your preparation.

Second, surround yourself with encouraging people. It can be helpful to find a study group, but be sure that the people you're around will encourage a positive attitude. If you spend time with others who are anxious or cynical, this will only contribute to your own anxiety. Look for others who are motivated to study hard from a desire to succeed, not from a fear of failure.

Third, reward yourself. A test is physically and mentally tiring, even without anxiety, and it can be helpful to have something to look forward to. Plan an activity following the test, regardless of the outcome, such as going to a movie or getting ice cream.

When you are taking the test, if you find yourself beginning to feel anxious, remind yourself that you know the material. Visualize successfully completing the test. Then take a few deep, relaxing breaths and return to it. Work through the questions carefully but with confidence, knowing that you are capable of succeeding.

Developing a healthy mental approach to test taking will also aid in other areas of life. Test anxiety affects more than just the actual test—it can be damaging to your mental health and even contribute to depression. It's important to beat test anxiety before it becomes a problem for more than testing.

Study Strategy

Being prepared for the test is necessary to combat anxiety, but what does being prepared look like? You may study for hours on end and still not feel prepared. What you need is a strategy for test prep. The next few pages outline our recommended steps to help you plan out and conquer the challenge of preparation.

Step 1: Scope Out the Test

Learn everything you can about the format (multiple choice, essay, etc.) and what will be on the test. Gather any study materials, course outlines, or sample exams that may be available. Not only will this help you to prepare, but knowing what to expect can help to alleviate test anxiety.

Step 2: Map Out the Material

Look through the textbook or study guide and make note of how many chapters or sections it has. Then divide these over the time you have. For example, if a book has 15 chapters and you have five days to study, you need to cover three chapters each day. Even better, if you have the time, leave an extra day at the end for overall review after you have gone through the material in depth.

If time is limited, you may need to prioritize the material. Look through it and make note of which sections you think you already have a good grasp on, and which need review. While you are studying, skim quickly through the familiar sections and take more time on the challenging parts.

Write out your plan so you don't get lost as you go. Having a written plan also helps you feel more in control of the study, so anxiety is less likely to arise from feeling overwhelmed at the amount to cover.

Step 3: Gather Your Tools

Decide what study method works best for you. Do you prefer to highlight in the book as you study and then go back over the highlighted portions? Or do you type out notes of the important information? Or is it helpful to make flashcards that you can carry with you? Assemble the pens, index cards, highlighters, post-it notes, and any other materials you may need so you won't be distracted by getting up to find things while you study.

If you're having a hard time retaining the information or organizing your notes, experiment with different methods. For example, try color-coding by subject with colored pens, highlighters, or post-it notes. If you learn better by hearing, try recording yourself reading your notes so you can listen while in the car, working out, or simply sitting at your desk. Ask a friend to quiz you from your flashcards, or try teaching someone the material to solidify it in your mind.

Step 4: Create Your Environment

It's important to avoid distractions while you study. This includes both the obvious distractions like visitors and the subtle distractions like an uncomfortable chair (or a too-comfortable couch that makes you want to fall asleep). Set up the best study environment possible: good lighting and a comfortable work area. If background music helps you focus, you may want to turn it on, but otherwise keep the room quiet. If you are using a computer to take notes, be sure you don't have any other windows open, especially applications like social media, games, or anything else that could distract you. Silence your phone and turn off notifications. Be sure to keep water close by so you stay hydrated while you study (but avoid unhealthy drinks and snacks).

Also, take into account the best time of day to study. Are you freshest first thing in the morning? Try to set aside some time then to work through the material. Is your mind clearer in the afternoon or evening? Schedule your study session then. Another method is to study at the same time of day that you will take the test, so that your brain gets used to working on the material at that time and will be ready to focus at test time.

Step 5: Study!

Once you have done all the study preparation, it's time to settle into the actual studying. Sit down, take a few moments to settle your mind so you can focus, and begin to follow your study plan. Don't give in to distractions or let yourself procrastinate. This is your time to prepare so you'll be ready to fearlessly approach the test. Make the most of the time and stay focused.

Of course, you don't want to burn out. If you study too long you may find that you're not retaining the information very well. Take regular study breaks. For example, taking five minutes out of every hour to walk briskly, breathing deeply and swinging your arms, can help your mind stay fresh.

As you get to the end of each chapter or section, it's a good idea to do a quick review. Remind yourself of what you learned and work on any difficult parts. When you feel that you've mastered the material, move on to the next part. At the end of your study session, briefly skim through your notes again.

But while review is helpful, cramming last minute is NOT. If at all possible, work ahead so that you won't need to fit all your study into the last day. Cramming overloads your brain with more information than it can process and retain, and your tired mind may struggle to recall even previously learned information when it is overwhelmed with last-minute study. Also, the urgent nature of cramming and the stress placed on your brain contribute to anxiety. You'll be more likely to go to the test feeling unprepared and having trouble thinking clearly.

So don't cram, and don't stay up late before the test, even just to review your notes at a leisurely pace. Your brain needs rest more than it needs to go over the information again. In fact, plan to finish your studies by noon or early afternoon the day before the test. Give your brain the rest of the day to relax or focus on other things, and get a good night's sleep. Then you will be fresh for the test and better able to recall what you've studied.

Step 6: Take a Practice Test

Many courses offer sample tests, either online or in the study materials. This is an excellent resource to check whether you have mastered the material, as well as to prepare for the test format and environment.

Check the test format ahead of time: the number of questions, the type (multiple choice, free response, etc.), and the time limit. Then create a plan for working through them. For example, if you have 30 minutes to take a 60-question test, your limit is 30 seconds per question. Spend less time on the questions you know well so that you can take more time on the difficult ones.

If you have time to take several practice tests, take the first one open book, with no time limit. Work through the questions at your own pace and make sure you fully understand them. Gradually work up to taking a test under test conditions: sit at a desk with all study materials put away and set a timer. Pace yourself to make sure you finish the test with time to spare and go back to check your answers if you have time.

After each test, check your answers. On the questions you missed, be sure you understand why you missed them. Did you misread the question (tests can use tricky wording)? Did you forget the information? Or was it something you hadn't learned? Go back and study any shaky areas that the practice tests reveal.

Taking these tests not only helps with your grade, but also aids in combating test anxiety. If you're already used to the test conditions, you're less likely to worry about it, and working through tests until you're scoring well gives you a confidence boost. Go through the practice tests until you feel comfortable, and then you can go into the test knowing that you're ready for it.

Test Tips

On test day, you should be confident, knowing that you've prepared well and are ready to answer the questions. But aside from preparation, there are several test day strategies you can employ to maximize your performance.

First, as stated before, get a good night's sleep the night before the test (and for several nights before that, if possible). Go into the test with a fresh, alert mind rather than staying up late to study.

Try not to change too much about your normal routine on the day of the test. It's important to eat a nutritious breakfast, but if you normally don't eat breakfast at all, consider eating just a protein bar. If you're a coffee drinker, go ahead and have your normal coffee. Just make sure you time it so that the caffeine doesn't wear off right in the middle of your test. Avoid sugary beverages, and drink enough water to stay hydrated but not so much that you need a restroom break 10 minutes into the test. If your test isn't first thing in the morning, consider going for a walk or doing a light workout before the test to get your blood flowing.

Allow yourself enough time to get ready, and leave for the test with plenty of time to spare so you won't have the anxiety of scrambling to arrive in time. Another reason to be early is to select a good seat. It's helpful to sit away from doors and windows, which can be distracting. Find a good seat, get out your supplies, and settle your mind before the test begins.

When the test begins, start by going over the instructions carefully, even if you already know what to expect. Make sure you avoid any careless mistakes by following the directions.

Then begin working through the questions, pacing yourself as you've practiced. If you're not sure on an answer, don't spend too much time on it, and don't let it shake your confidence. Either skip it and come back later, or eliminate as many wrong answers as possible and guess among the remaining ones. Don't dwell on these questions as you continue—put them out of your mind and focus on what lies ahead.

Be sure to read all of the answer choices, even if you're sure the first one is the right answer. Sometimes you'll find a better one if you keep reading. But don't second-guess yourself if you do immediately know the answer. Your gut instinct is usually right. Don't let test anxiety rob you of the information you know.

If you have time at the end of the test (and if the test format allows), go back and review your answers. Be cautious about changing any, since your first instinct tends to be correct, but make sure you didn't misread any of the questions or accidentally mark the wrong answer choice. Look over any you skipped and make an educated guess.

At the end, leave the test feeling confident. You've done your best, so don't waste time worrying about your performance or wishing you could change anything. Instead, celebrate the successful completion of this test. And finally, use this test to learn how to deal with anxiety even better next time.

Review Video: Test Anxiety
Visit mometrix.com/academy and enter code: 100340

Important Qualification

Not all anxiety is created equal. If your test anxiety is causing major issues in your life beyond the classroom or testing center, or if you are experiencing troubling physical symptoms related to your anxiety, it may be a sign of a serious physiological or psychological condition. If this sounds like your situation, we strongly encourage you to seek professional help.

Online Resources

Due to our efforts to try to keep this book to a manageable length, we've created a link that will give you access to all of your online resources:

mometrix.com/resources719/chfm

It's Your Moment, Let's Celebrate It!

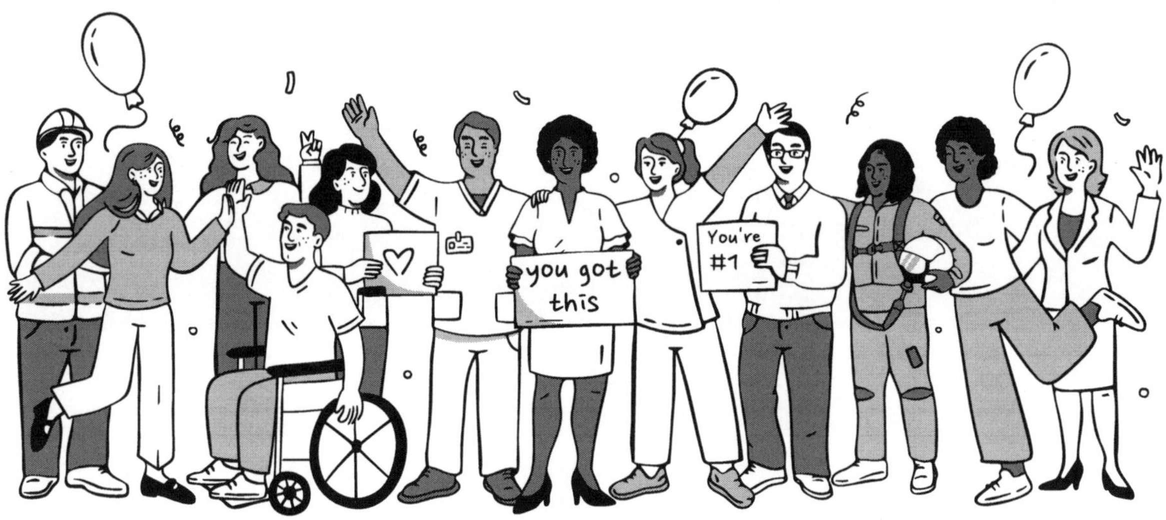

Share your story @mometrixtestpreparation